The
Organic Food
Handbook

A Consumer's Guide to Buying and Eating Organic Food

KEN ROSEBORO

Basic
Health
PUBLICATIONS, INC.

The information contained in this book is based upon the research and personal and professional experiences of the author. It is not intended as a substitute for consulting with your physician or other healthcare provider. Any attempt to diagnose and treat an illness should be done under the direction of a healthcare professional.

The publisher does not advocate the use of any particular healthcare protocol but believes the information in this book should be available to the public. The publisher and author are not responsible for any adverse effects or consequences resulting from the use of the suggestions, preparations, or procedures discussed in this book. Should the reader have any questions concerning the appropriateness of any procedures or preparation mentioned, the author and the publisher strongly suggest consulting a professional healthcare advisor.

Basic Health Guides are published by
Basic Health Publications, Inc.
28812 Top of the World Drive
Laguna Beach, CA 92651
949-715-7327 • www.basichealthpub.com

Library of Congress Cataloging-in-Publication Data

Roseboro, Ken
    The organic food handbook : a consumer's guide to buying and eating organic food / by Ken Roseboro.
        p. cm.
    Includes bibliographical references and index.
    ISBN-13: 978-1-59120-159-5
    ISBN-10: 1-59120-159-4
    1. Nutrition. 2. Health. 3. Organic farming. 4. Natural foods.
5. Natural foods—Purchasing. I. Title.

    RA784.R655   2006
    641.3′02—dc22

                                        2006004490

Editor: Thomas Hirsch • Typesetting/Book design: Gary A. Rosenberg
Series Cover Design: Mike Stromberg

Printed in the United States of America

10   9   8   7   6   5   4   3   2

CONTENTS

For Mirjana
and her unbounded love,
support, and devotion

EDITOR'S NOTE

Dear Reader,

Welcome to the *Basic Earth Guide* series! As you know, the natural world is becoming degraded at an alarming rate. Hardly a day passes without a new headline about the effects of global warming, species loss, and other distressing environmental news. Incredibly, during every second of every day, more than an acre of the world's precious and irreplaceable rain forests is being lost. The depletion of beneficial oxygen-producing plants, which are part of the rain forest's ecosystem, makes us vulnerable to the 6,000 metric tons of carbon dioxide emitted into the atmosphere each year. The subtraction of oxygen, and the addition of carbon dioxide, adversely affects everyone's health and quality of life. This example is but one of a number of environmental problems that beset us. Residues of toxic pollutants, ranging from pesticides in our food; chemicals in our homes such as cleaning agents, sealants, solvents, formaldehyde, and lead-contaminated paint; gas leakages from cooking stoves; gases from plastics; fragrances in consumer products; to a host of other volatile substances, both indoors and outdoors, affect our health. Over time, chronic exposures to these substances compromise our immune systems and contribute to various illnesses and health problems. Some experts caution that *we have only one generation of time to reverse conditions in our polluted environment, or we shall experience irreversible damage.* Many people feel that the problems are on such a vast scale, are so complex and overwhelming, that the individual's efforts are futile. They are wrong.

The *Basic Earth Guide* series demonstrates that you, as an individual, can take meaningful action. Each *Basic Earth Guide* sets forth a group of ecological problems you face daily, and provides alternative environmentally sound practical solutions. Each *Basic Earth Guide* provides the best researched ideas, and up-to-date information, to help you transform your day-to-day living into an ecologically sounder environment. The works are written simply and lucidly for easy comprehension. Among topics covered are renewable energy, "green" building and retrofitting, home care and maintenance, personal care products, and ecological lifestyles.

As a reader of *Basic Earth Guides,* you will become better informed and motivated to improve the environmental quality of your life, as well as for those around you. There can be a new world out there! We thank you for allowing us to introduce it to you.

Green regards,
Tom Hirsch, series editor

P.S. Do let us know about additional subjects that interest you, for us to consider as future *Basic Earth Guides.* You can reach us at ngoldfind@basicmediagroup.com.

INTRODUCTION

The way food is grown, produced, and eaten in the United States and around the world is changing. The conventional, industrial system of producing food, while efficient at producing mass quantities, is increasingly inefficient and creating big problems. Americans are becoming obese due to poor diets; foodborne illnesses are increasing; the nutrition of fruits and vegetables is decreasing; pesticides sprayed on food crops are sickening farm workers and polluting groundwater; inhumane poultry, hog, and cattle "factory farms" pollute air and water and create antibiotic-resistant bacteria; and genetically engineered crops pose great risks to human health and the environment. It's not a pretty picture.

As a result, more and more people want a healthier alternative to conventional food. They want food produced without pesticides, antibiotics, hormones, and genetic engineering. They want food that benefits human health and preserves the environment. They want fresh food grown locally by family farmers. The food these people are choosing is organic.

COMMON SENSE

Once derided as a hippie fad, organic is the fastest growing segment of the United States food industry, with consumer demand increasing by nearly 20 percent each year.

Many people choose organic for a simple reason: common sense. It makes sense that food produced without toxic chemicals, sewage sludge, and risky genetic engineering would be healthier and better for the environment. It makes sense that organic food produced and sold by local farmers is fresher and tastes better than conventional supermarket food transported thousands of miles. It makes sense that building fertile soils, a primary goal of organic farming, would produce healthy plants that would in turn create nutritious food. In contrast, industrial farming's chemical-intensive methods degrade soils, producing foods of questionable nutritional value.

CONCISE, SIMPLE GUIDE

This handbook provides a concise, simple guide to organic food. It helps you understand what organic food is, how it is produced, why more and more people are choosing it, why it presently costs more than conventional food, and why it is a better choice for you, your family, and the world.

The handbook aims to give you the big picture of organic food. You'll see why organic is not just a fad but a growing movement that is fundamentally changing our food for the better. You'll understand how certification ensures that organic food is produced to the highest standards, and why local organic is even better than organic. You'll see how the organic community must fight corporate and government attempts to weaken these high standards. You'll learn about research demonstrating the benefits of organic food to human health and the environment. You'll meet "organic heroes," the dedicated people who are committed to providing the highest quality foods, and learn how to buy organic foods at the best prices. Finally, the book aims to help you realize that by choosing organic you can make a positive difference in the world. Organic is, as research is beginning to show, a healthier choice for you and your family. But the impact of choosing organic extends beyond your life, rippling out to support family farms and rural communities; it also promotes healthy soil, clean air and water, and preserves biodiversity. As American poet, philosopher and farmer Wendell Berry said, "How we eat determines to a considerable extent how the world is used."

Chapter 1

ORGANIC GOES MAINSTREAM

There is here and abroad, a slow, incremental, but ineluctable
movement toward food that nourishes both person and place,
that is grown with a far richer knowledge and awareness
of biology than can be found in the five-gallon cans of
chlorinated hydrocarbons provided by Shell or Uniroyal.

—Paul Hawken, author of *Natural Capitalism:*
Creating the Next Industrial Revolution

An Acme supermarket in suburban Westmont, New Jersey, looks like most other supermarkets in the United States. Bright, spacious, and clean with long aisles filled with thousands of foods, fresh to frozen. Yet, even here in a suburban supermarket, one can't help but notice a growing trend in the foods that Americans eat. There are new sections of the store with signs reading "Organic Produce." There are old, familiar brand names—Dole, Heinz, and Frito-Lay—on new, organic products, such as lettuce, ketchup, and corn chips. This Acme store—along with thousands of supermarkets nationwide—is displaying many more foods labeled "organic."

Once considered a counterculture fad of the 1960s and 1970s, organic foods have gone mainstream. Organic is a growing movement that is fundamentally changing the way food is grown, produced, and eaten in the United States and around the world. Organic provides a viable, life-supporting alternative to industrialized agriculture, whose methods are damaging human health, polluting the environment, and eroding soils.

An increasing number of people eat organic foods because they want pure, healthy, and safe foods produced without chemical pesticides and fertilizers, artificial hormones, antibiotics, and genetically engineered ingredients. They eat organic because they see it as a healthier option for their families, and one that tastes better. Organic consumers want foods that foster a cleaner environment and support family farmers.

WHAT IS ORGANIC?

According to the National Organic Standards Board, which oversees organic food production in the United States, organic "is a labeling term that denotes products produced under the authority of the Organic Foods Production Act. The principal guidelines for organic production are to use materials and practices that enhance the ecological balance of natural systems and that integrate the parts of the farming system into an ecological whole."

Furthermore, organic is much more than the absence of chemicals and synthetic products; it is a synergy joining soil, plants, the farmer, community, and the environment into a living food production system. Each stage of the system supports and benefits the following stage.

Organic farmers work with nature to produce food, as opposed to overwhelming it with chemicals. They enhance soil fertility using compost, cover crops, and manures, aiming to strengthen plants' natural ability to withstand pests and weeds. They use beneficial insects and natural, environmentally safe methods to limit pests. They use mulch to limit weeds and alternate crop plantings each year to preserve the soil, break weed and insect lifecycles, and add nutrients, instead of relying on chemical fertilizers. They breed seed varieties to adapt to local growing conditions and to resist insects and disease. Finally, organic farmers rely on their intelligence and experience working with nature and utilize its processes to produce healthy food.

Again, according to the National Organic Standards Board, "The primary goal of organic agriculture is to optimize the health and productivity of interdependent communities of soil life, plants, animals and people."

ORGANIC CERTIFICATION

The most visible sign of organic's mainstream status is the green and white "USDA Organic" seal found on organic foods. The seal indicates that a product has been certified according to strict standards established by the U.S. National Organic Program. The standards prohibit chemical pesticides and fertilizers, genetically engineered ingredients, antibiotics, and artificial hormones. Also prohibited are irradiation, sewage sludge, and other synthetic "inputs" and ingredients. Certification assures consumers that products labeled organic meet high standards for safety, quality, and purity.

MORE THAN FRUITS AND VEGETABLES

In the past, the term "organic" may have created images of granola-crunching hippies or wilted and bruised produce sold in natural food stores. Those days are gone. Today's organic fruits and vegetables don't look wilted or bruised. They are diverse in unique varieties and brim with freshness, delicious flavor, and health-enhancing vitamins, minerals, and antioxidants.

At the Westmont Acme supermarket, a special organic produce section features apples, carrots, cucumbers, lettuce, oranges, peppers, and zucchinis to name a few. But there is much more than fruit and vegetables. Virtually every aisle in the store contains organic food products, including baby foods, cereals, chicken and vegetable broths, cookies, corn chips, macaroni and cheese, pasta, pretzels, rice, tofu, salad dressing, soymilk, sugar, tomato juice, and more.

In the past, supermarkets placed organic foods into a special "Natural Foods" section. Today, organic foods are found on the same shelves with conventional brands. At the Acme store, Heinz organic ketchup, Tostitos organic corn tortilla chips, Swanson organic chicken broth, and Domino organic sugar are right next to their conventional counterparts.

Other familiar brands featuring organic products include Dole, Campbell's and Gerber. There are familiar organic products such as Newman's Own Organics cookies, Eden Foods pasta and soymilk, Nature's Path cereals, and Stonyfield Farms milk and yogurt.

Still, the wide range of organic products found at Acme represents only the tip of the iceberg. There are also beef, beer, chicken, chocolates, frozen foods, turkey, wines, and even pet foods. And these are just the food items customers can check off their shopping lists. There are organic personal care products, such as shampoos, soaps, and household cleaning products. Organic cotton clothing is also popular.

The top-selling organic food products are fruits and vegetables, dairy products, beverages, breads and grain-based products, prepared and packaged foods, snacks and desserts, and meat and poultry.

FASTEST GROWING SEGMENT OF FOOD INDUSTRY

All these organic products are appearing on store shelves because a growing number of people are buying them. According to the Hartman Group, a market research firm, nearly 75 percent of American consumers say they use organic products at least occasionally. Organic is the fastest-growing segment of the American food industry. Sales of organic products in the United States reached $14.0 billion in 2005 and are projected to reach $30 billion by 2007. Despite the growth, organic food sales account for just 2.5 percent of food sales in the United States.

Certified organic farm acreage in the United States doubled between 1997 and 2003, growing from more than 1 million acres to 2.2 million acres and 8,035 certified organic farms. As with food sales, organic acreage accounts for a small fraction, 0.4 percent, of total United States cropland.

A 2005 survey by natural food retailer Whole Foods Market found that nearly two-thirds of Americans, 65 percent, have tried organic foods and beverages, and one in ten use organic products regularly or several times per week.

Another indication of the growth of the organic industry is the success of natural food chains Whole Foods Market and Wild Oats Markets. Whole Foods has 180 supermarket-size stores in North America and the United Kingdom with 32,000 employees. Wild Oats, which started with one store in Boulder, Colorado, in 1987, now operates 110 stores in the United States and Canada.

The strong growth of the organic industry has attracted large, mainstream food companies. Coca Cola, Frito-Lay, General Mills, Kellogg Company, H.J. Heinz, Proctor & Gamble, Quaker Oats, and Kraft Foods have either launched organic brands or purchased organic food companies. The organic community is divided over "Big Organic." Some say the big names will increase acceptance of organic foods and expand the market even more, while others believe the companies may try to weaken the strict standards that have been the hallmark of organic production.

The extent to which organic foods have become mainstream is seen at supermarkets such as Acme. In fact, nearly half of consumers that purchase natural and organic foods buy them in traditional supermarkets. This is because large food companies can place their organic products into established distribution channels with supermarket chains. In addition, supermarket chains such as Hy-Vee, Safeway, Kroger, Giant, Publix, and Price Chopper have launched their own organic brands.

Suprisingly, the biggest seller of organic foods may soon be Wal-Mart. The retail giant has made a strong commitment to organic and plans to stock several hundred organic products in its stores. Other retail giants such as Target and Costco also sell organic foods.

People can buy organic foods at many other venues. Restaurants serving organic range from fast food at retail chains such as O'Naturals in New England and Organic to Go on the West Coast to upscale "slow food" at cafes such as Le Pain Quotidien in New York City and Restaurant Nora in Washington, D.C. Major league baseball stadiums in St. Louis and San Diego now sell organic hot dogs. Organic foods are served in restaurants at Yellowstone, Yosemite, and other national parks; Niagara Falls State Park; and the Kennedy Space Center Visitor Complex. Even fast-food giant McDonald's serves organic coffee at 650 of its restaurants in New England. Many schools, colleges, and universities, including Stanford, Princeton, the University of Wisconsin, Colorado College, Oberlin College in Ohio, and Maharishi University of Management in Iowa, serve organic foods to their students.

In addition, a strong local foods movement has emerged nationwide as evidenced by the growing popularity of farmers markets and community-supported agriculture. These direct, farmer-to-consumer programs allow people to buy local, fresh organic foods at lower prices, while supporting small family farms.

WHY ARE PEOPLE EATING ORGANIC?

People are buying organic foods for a variety of reasons, with health being at the top of the list. A 2002 study by the Food Marketing Institute (FMI) and *Prevention* magazine found that more than 60 percent of American shoppers believe that organic foods are better for their health. According to the Whole Foods Market survey, Americans buy organic to avoid pesticides, and because they think organic is fresher and better for their health. In addition, 52.4 percent of survey respondents say organic foods are better for the environment, and 57 percent believe organics are better for supporting small and local farmers. Nearly one-third believes organic products taste better, and 42 percent say organic foods are better quality than conventional foods.

Organic foods are seen as healthier because, unlike conventional foods, they are produced without chemicals or genetic engineering. Scientific research is exposing the health hazards of chemical pesticides. Genetically engineered foods, which permeate the food supply, raise possible health risks. Eating organic is one of the best ways to avoid the hazards of both.

A growing body of research confirms the wisdom of eating organic. Several studies show that organic foods contain significantly fewer pesticide residues than conventional foods. Preliminary research comparing the nutritional value of organic and conventional foods finds that organic foods contain higher amounts of vitamins, minerals, and cancer-fighting antioxidants.

MYTHS AND REALITIES ABOUT ORGANIC BUYERS

Organic's arrival as mainstream is evidenced by the fact that people who buy organic represent all ages, backgrounds, income and education levels, and ethnic groups. One myth about organic foods is that they are purchased by highly educated, wealthy Caucasians only. The research that has come in from the Hartman Group reveals organic buyers are much more diverse. In reality, minority Americans—Asian, Native, Hispanic, and African are more likely to buy organic than Caucasians. Laurie Demeritt, president of the Hartman Group states, "We see purchase and use of organics by a cross-section of the population representative of nearly all consumers."

Organic consumers do tend to be more educated. However, the Hartman Group found that 41.8 percent of organic consumers have annual incomes of less than $40,000, demonstrating that organic foods are not a luxury of the rich. People buy organic foods based on the food's perceived value as being healthier rather than as a luxury item they can afford.

As a result of fast-growing acceptance among a wide range of consumers, Demeritt says organic food is much more than a niche market for specialized consumers. "There is a clear divergence of consumer values, attitudes, and interests with respect to organic," she says.

Another myth debunked by the Hartman Group study is that price is the main reason why most consumers do not buy organic foods. In reality, consumers do not buy organic foods because they had never considered them before. The study also found that a seeming lack of availability is another reason why people don't buy organic. For example, shoppers at Acme shop out of habit and may not go out of their way to look for organic products. As a result, the Hartman Group recommends that supermarkets place organic foods on shelves with other products and not in special sections, which Acme and other supermarkets now do.

THE BIG PICTURE

The mainstreaming of organic is not limited to the United States. Globally, the market for organic foods is now more than $23 billion and growing, according to *Organic Monitor*. Western Europe is the second leading market for organic foods with nearly $10 billion in sales. Worldwide acreage of organic crops now tops 59 million in 100 countries. Australia leads the world with 24 million acres, followed by Argentina with 6.2 million, Italy with 2.4 million, and then the United States with 2.2 million. However, the United States ranks thirty-sixth among all nations in percentage of agricultural land for organic use.

Chapter 2

REAPING
DESTRUCTION

*This is the end result of a factory-farm system that appears as a living,
continental-scale monument to Rube Goldberg, a black-mass remake of the
loaves-and-fishes miracle. Prairie's productivity is lost for grain, grain's
productivity is lost in livestock, livestock's protein is lost to human fat—
all federally subsidized for about $15 billion a year.*

—Richard Manning, from *The Oil We Eat:
Following the Food Chain Back to Iraq*

Bill McCracken and his family have taken a novel approach to farming in rural Iowa: They grow food for human consumption. Surrounding the McCracken's Choice Earth Farm in Brighton, Iowa, are vast fields of corn and soybeans, mostly grown for animal feed, stretching as far as the eye can see. Choice Earth Farm looks much like the neighboring farms, with open fields, farmhouse, grain silos, barns, and cows, but the McCrackens have gone against current farming practices to renew an age-old tradition that has nearly disappeared in Iowa. Instead of growing "monocultures" of corn and soybeans as the neighboring farms do, Choice Earth grows vegetables. Instead of using industrial farming methods—chemical pesticides, fertilizers, and genetically engineered crops—Choice Earth grows food organically. Instead of a massive "factory" farm operated by tenant farmers, Choice Earth is a small family farm, owned and operated by McCracken and his two daughters, Jocelyn and Alisha and their husbands.

The McCrackens, and a growing number of farmers, have switched to organic because they believe it is a healthier, more sustainable alternative to conventional farming, whose methods are increasingly seen as a threat to human health and the environment.

INDUSTRIAL AGRICULTURE

Most foods sold in supermarkets are produced using a system of industrialized agriculture whose methods have evolved since the mid-1900s. During this time, the principles of industrialization, with its emphases on mass-production, mechanization, efficiency, and simplification, were applied to agriculture. New labor-saving farm machinery, such as the tractor, combine, and cultivator, allowed farms to increase in size. Small family farms gave way to larger corporate-owned "factory farms." Chemicals developed as weapons during the Second World War, such as ammonium nitrate and organophosphate nerve gas, were reinvented as fertilizers and pesticides for agriculture. A "Green Revolution" created high-yielding seeds that promised to end hunger. While the new seeds did increase agricultural production, the Green Revolution did not end hunger, it actually reduced the variety of crops produced. As a result, agricultural production narrowed to millions of acres of crop "monocultures," such as corn, soybeans, and wheat that require intensive use of chemical pesticides and fertilizers.

"AS YOU SOW, SO SHALL YOU REAP"

Industrial agriculture views nature, including soil, plants, and insects, as something to control and kill, if necessary. Soil and plants receive heavy doses of nitrogen "fixes" to stimulate growth. Farmers use highly toxic pesticides to kill weeds, insects, and fungi. Age-old agricultural practices, such as crop rotations to build soil fertility and reduce pests, have been ignored, replaced by chemical "inputs." Cattle, hogs, and chickens are crammed into concentrated animal feeding operations (CAFOs) and heavily treated with antibiotics, which can later contaminate water sources and vegetables, posing a threat to human health. The vital connection between farmers and people who buy their crops has been severed. Food has become a highly processed, slick-packaged commodity eaten by "consumers."

Subjugating and poisoning nature is bound to cause negative repercussions. Today the world reaps catastrophic problems, including foodborne illnesses, "Mad Cow" disease, polluted water supplies, depleted soils, and loss of crop diversity and wildlife.

Foodborne Illnesses

Over the last thirty years, foodborne illnesses have increased tenfold. Each year, there are an estimated 76 million cases of foodborne disease resulting in 325,000 hospitalizations and 5,000 deaths, according to the World Health Organization.

Foodborne diseases are caused by pathogens, such as the E. coli 0157:H7 bacterium. But the Centers for Disease Control and Prevention (CDC) estimates that more than three-fourths of food-related illnesses and deaths in the United States are caused by infectious agents that have not yet been identified. In his best-selling book *Fast Food Nation*, Eric Schlosser describes how the United States' meat processing industry, with huge feedlots and slaughterhouses, has created conditions for outbreaks of foodborne illnesses that can potentially sicken millions of people. Only thirteen meatpacking houses slaughter most of the beef in the United States. In such a centralized system, there is much greater potential for meat tainted with pathogens to be distributed, sold, and consumed far and wide. Several incidents underscore the kinds of problems that can occur. In 1993, 700 people in five states got sick eating hamburgers sold at Jack in the Box restaurants. Two hundred were hospitalized and four died. In 1998, tainted hot dogs sickened scores of people, killing 15.

Fast Food Nation focuses on the negative health, social, and environmental impacts of fast-food restaurants in America. Schlosser details horrific working conditions in meatpacking facilities, feedlots holding thousands of cattle wallowing in manure and disease, and chemical-intensive French fry production from farming to flavoring.

Antibiotics and Hormones

Beef cattle and hogs are given hormones and antibiotics to stimulate growth. The heavy use of antibiotics in farm animals is creating antibiotic-resistant pathogens, a major threat to human health because pathogens could render medicinal antibiotics ineffective.

A study published in the *Journal of Environmental Quality* found that antibiotics given to farm animals could end up in vegetables. Researchers found that corn, cabbage, and onions absorbed the antibiotic chlortetracycline from the manure of pigs given the antibiotic and used as fertilizer.

Ingesting antibiotics can cause bacteria naturally present in the intestinal tract, including disease-causing bacteria, to become drug-resistant. It is interesting to note that while the application of manure for fertilizer is unregulated in conventional farming, organic standards set strict guidelines, such as composting, for the application of manure on organic fields.

Dairy cows are injected with genetically engineered bovine growth hormone (rBGH) to increase milk production. Consumer groups say milk from cows treated with rBGH contains high levels of insulin growth factor-1, a promoter of tumor growth. The controversial hormone was banned in Canada and Europe.

Mad Cow

Industrial agriculture has given the world bovine spongiform encephalopathy (BSE), better known as mad cow disease, a fatal, brain-wasting disease in cattle. Mad cow, first discovered in Great Britain in 1986, resulted when cows ate contaminated feed made from rendered cattle brains, blood, fat, and bone meal, essentially turning the cows into cannibals. People eating meat from the diseased animals contracted a similar fatal, brain-wasting disease called Creutzfeldt-Jakob disease (CJD). Both diseases, which have no cure, involve proteins called prions that eat sponge-like holes in brains. About 100 people have died from CJD, mostly in Great Britain.

In addition to 180,000 confirmed cases of mad cow in Britain, the disease has spread to other European countries, Argentina, Canada, Japan, and the United States, mainly as a result of Britain exporting the contaminated feed.

Eric Schlosser believes the United States, which continues to allow beef producers to use rendered animal parts as feed, is vulnerable to an outbreak of mad cow. Government regulators are not looking hard to find it. Of 375 million cattle slaughtered between 1990 and 2001, only 15,000 were tested for mad cow.

John Stauber, author of *Mad Cow USA,* says, "The U.S. mad cow testing system seems designed to cover up mad cow disease rather than find it."

Corn and Obesity

Corn is king in American agriculture, grown on more than 80 million acres each year. Several experts link the over-production of corn to America's obesity epidemic, which causes 400,000 deaths per year and increases the risk of heart disease, diabetes, and cancer. Corn is processed into feed and food ingredients, such as corn syrup and high fructose corn syrup. These cheap sweeteners have replaced sugar in soft drinks and other products and have allowed food companies to "supersize" portions without reducing profits.

Michael Pollan, food writer and author of the *Botany of Desire*, says the switch to corn sweeteners in the 1980s corresponds exactly to the beginning of the obesity epidemic and type 2 diabetes in the United States. Dr. George A. Bray, an obesity researcher and professor of medicine at Louisiana State University Medical Center, agrees, calling the connection "a very, very striking relationship."

Pesticide Threats

Industrial agriculture relies on toxic pesticides, including insecticides, herbicides, and fungicides, and their use is making people sick and polluting the environment. A 2001 United States government study states, "Exposure to pesticides can cause a range of ill effects in humans, from relatively mild effects such as headaches, fatigue, and nausea, to more serious effects such as cancer and neurological disorders."

Pesticide residues are pervasive, found in the air, soil, water, food, and our bodies. A report by the Environmental Illness Society of Canada states, "Once released into the environment, the spread of pesticides cannot be controlled."

The hazards of pesticides are discussed in greater detail in Chapter 6, but suffice to say pesticides pose a major threat to human health and the environment.

Less Nutritious Food

A University of Texas study published in the *Journal of the American College of Nutrition* found that the nutrient value of forty-three common vegetables and fruits has declined over the past fifty years. Levels of essential nutrients, including protein, calcium, phosphorus, iron, riboflavin, and ascorbic acid, have declined between 6 and 38 percent, raising significant questions about how modern agriculture practices are affecting food crops.

Environmental Damage

One would assume that rural areas with open spaces and farms would be cleaner, less polluted places to live than urban areas. Not true. Pesticides from farms drift in the air, permeate the soil, and leech into drinking water. The air near large hog farms and cattle feedlots reeks with toxic gases and the stench of manure, which seeps into water supplies. Crop monocultures of corn, soybeans, wheat, and cotton, which cover 82 percent of America's farmland, have eliminated agricultural diversity, eroded soils, and rendered them lifeless from heavy chemical use.

Industrial agriculture's damage to the environment and wildlife continues to mount:

- Nearly one-third of the world's arable land has been lost to erosion and continues to be lost at a rate of more than 24,000 acres per year.

- Each spring, runoff of chemical fertilizers from Midwestern farms into the Mississippi River reduces oxygen levels in large areas of the Gulf of Mexico, killing sea plants and animals. This hypoxia creates a "dead zone" about the size of New Jersey.

- An estimated 67 million birds die each year as a result of pesticide use on farmland.

- In a study published in *Science,* University of Minnesota scientists concluded that continued expansion of industrial farming "has the potential to have massive, irreversible environmental impacts," degrade biodiversity, and expose humans to markedly higher levels of pesticides.

Food Waste

Industrial agriculture is also inefficient. Research by Timothy Jones, an anthropologist at the University of Arizona, found that 50 percent of all food produced in the United States goes to waste, a $43 billion loss per year. Jones estimates that cutting food waste by half could reduce negative environmental impacts by 25 percent through reduced landfills, less soil depletion, and fewer applications of chemical fertilizers and pesticides.

"Pig Prisons"

Something else besides corn and soybeans is sprouting on Midwestern farms: hog confinement buildings. Known technically as concentrated animal feeding operations (CAFOs), but perhaps more accurately as "pig prisons," these buildings house anywhere from a few hundred to several thousand hogs in tiny pens.

Scientists from the Universities of Iowa and North Carolina found that people living near large hog farms reported health problems, including respiratory illness, headaches, depression, diarrhea, and nausea caused by air emissions from the facilities.

A tragic example is Bob Thornell of Paulding, Ohio, who lost his health, home, and job as a result of a large hog farm near his forty-acre farm. During the late 1990s and early 2000s, the stench of manure and hydrogen sulfide gas emitting from manure pits caused brain damage to Thornell and his wife, Diane, forcing them to move from their home. Thornell's health got so bad that he had to quit his teaching job.

CAFOs contribute to the 1.3 billion tons of animal waste produced each year in the United States—five tons for every American citizen. A "small" CAFO holding 2,400 hogs produces a million gallons of manure each year. Runoff from such factory farms is the major polluter of United States waterways.

Genetic Engineering as a "Solution"

As evidence of industrial agriculture's hazards mount, agricultural experts say that genetically engineered crops will reduce pesticide use and "feed the world." It is ironic that chemical companies, who developed destructive pesticides and fertilizers, now claim that their genetically engineered crops will help solve the problems that their pesticides created.

The reality is genetic engineering, a risky technology that involves splicing together genes from bacteria and other species into plants is likely to create even greater destruction. Manipulating DNA, the building block of life, can create new allergens and toxins in foods and poses environmental hazards, such as the creation of "superweeds" and the killing of monarch butterflies.

SOCIAL IMPACTS

Industrial agriculture drives family farmers out of business. Farmers make less and less money due to low prices for corn, soybeans, and wheat, forcing them to "get big or get out." Many chose the latter. Prior to the industrialization of agriculture, there were 7 million American farmers. Today, there are about 2 million even though the population has doubled. From 1997 to 2002, Iowa lost 22 percent of its midsize farms. The loss of family farms kills rural communities. "We are in danger of losing our human capital in farming," says Fred Kirschenmann, director of the Leopold Center for Sustainable Agriculture at Iowa State University. On the other hand, as we will see in the next chapter, organic farming helps family farms thrive, keeping rural communities vital.

Industrial agriculture is propped up by more than $20 billion dollars in government subsidies, paid each year mostly to large agribusiness companies and paid for by American taxpayers. These agribusiness giants, who dominate food production, exert increasing control over the government to relax regulations on pesticides, genetically modified crops, testing of meat for mad cow disease, and other food safety measures.

ORGANIC ALTERNATIVE

Against this background of illness, obesity, pollution, and corporate hegemony, it is no wonder that more and more consumers want organic foods, and that the McCracken family chose to grow them. "Organic has a lot of potential to take off," says Jocelyn McCracken, who has a master's degree in chemistry.

Unlike people leaving family farms, Jocelyn and her husband, Tim Engman, returned after living in Chicago. Ironically, Engman worked for Pharmacia, a company that owned Monsanto, the major developer of genetically engineered crops.

The McCrackens converted their 110-acre farm to organic production and launched Choice Earth Farms, a community supported agriculture (CSA) program. Farmers operating a CSA program sell membership shares to people in neighboring communities in return for delivering fresh produce. As a result, the McCrackens are paid directly by members without a middleman, while members receive fresh local produce each week throughout the growing season.

In contrast to their neighbors who grow thousands of acres of corn and soybeans, Choice Earth Farms grows sweet corn and lots of vegetables, including beets, broccoli, carrots, cauliflower, cucumbers, eggplant, lettuce, okra, onions, peppers, radishes, turnips, several varieties of tomatoes, and more. Many of these are heirloom varieties that have been passed down from generation to generation.

Choice Earth Farms uses no pesticides, chemical fertilizers, or genetically engineered crops—practices prohibited by organic farming standards. Walking through his farm, Bill McCracken reaches down, picks a broccoli shoot, and eats it. Try doing that on an industrial farm doused with pesticides.

Instead of fertilizers, the McCrackens plant "green manures," such as alfalfa and clover to build soil fertility. "The secret to success in organic farming is soil fertility. The better prepared the soil is, the better it will produce," says Bill, who earned an agronomy degree at Iowa State University.

Most important, the McCrackens believe they are helping to reestablish the vital food link between farmers and families. "People have lost sight of what our food chain is. We are reeducating people to understand what good, local food tastes like," says Jocelyn. "I'd like to see all of Iowa become a CSA."

Chapter 3

THE WISDOM
OF ORGANIC

*In the final analysis, the only true dependable production technologies are
those that are sustainable over the long term. By that very definition, they
must avoid erosion, pollution, environmental degradation, and resource
waste. Any rational food-production system will emphasize the well-being
of the soil-air-water biosphere, the creatures which inhabit it,
and the human beings who depend on it.*

—Eliot Coleman, writing in *The New Organic Grower*

No one works more closely with nature than farmers, particularly
organic farmers. Organic farmers have a deep appreciation for
and seek to understand nature's life-sustaining processes, aiming to
work in harmony with them to produce healthy food. They possess a
long-term perspective, wanting to produce a positive, lasting impact
on the environment, communities, and human health for future generations. As they culture food crops, organic farmers culture within
themselves a down-to-earth sensibility along with a spiritual perspective about nature's greater intelligence.

THE JOURNEY OF AN ORGANIC FARMER

A good example is David Vetter, owner of Grain Place Foods, based in
Marquette, Nebraska. Vetter has grown organic grains for more than
thirty years. His father, Don, also a farmer, instilled the values of
organic farming in his son. The elder Vetter stopped using agricultural
chemicals in the early 1950s when his neighbors were just starting.

David chose the path of an organic farmer at a time when no one
in his area did. He was, as he says, "a topic of coffee shop conversation" among skeptical neighboring farmers who said he wouldn't last
farming organically. Even children of conventional farmers ridiculed
David's children about organic farming.

Vetter tried many crops that failed to find a few that succeeded. He carved out markets for organic soybeans and popcorn where none existed, financed a processing facility on a vision, and put his family farm on the line to make it a reality.

Despite the challenges, Vetter succeeded because of his long-term commitment, looking, as he says, at the impact of his work on the land 100 years ahead. He succeeded with good stewardship of the land, his willingness to teach and help other organic farmers, and his desire to produce wholesome organic grains.

Today, Vetter remains humble. He is not entirely joking when he says, "We're still in transition to organic."

SYNTHESIS OF OLD AND NEW

Organic agriculture, also known as "regenerative," "biological," or "ecological" agriculture, falls under the larger category of sustainable agriculture, which aims to produce food in a way that will "sustain" natural resources and human life for future generations.

Sustainable agriculture practices cover a broad spectrum, ranging from low-input, reduced-chemical and chemical-free practices to organic and biodynamic agriculture. The latter system combines traditional organic farming techniques with practices that seek to adapt a farm to natural rhythms of the sun and moon and to increase the vital life force or energy described in mystical traditions. Organic farming is considered by many to be a new alternative to so-called conventional farming described in Chapter 2. In reality, organic is the oldest system of farming in the world, while chemical-based industrial farming has developed over the last fifty years.

Most important, modern organic agriculture is not a return to the past but a synthesis of tried-and-true and innovative agricultural practices. The result is an efficient, economically viable, and sustainable system to produce healthy food. While employing age-old techniques, such as crop rotations and composting, organic farmers readily adopt new technologies and techniques, such as more efficient tools and machinery and new crop varieties, ever seeking ways to improve production.

Innovation is key to organic farming, even if the new solutions sometimes fail. "If you're going to be an organic farmer," says David Vetter. "You have to be willing to make big mistakes by the highway where everyone can see."

FERTILE SOIL IS KEY

The National Organic Standards Board's definition of organic states, "Organic agriculture is an ecological production management system that promotes and enhances biodiversity, biological cycles and soil biological activity."

The key to organic farming lies in enhancing soil biological activity and thus its fertility. Steve Gillman, an organic farmer in New York, states, "Fertile soil has the capacity to resist and suppress pests and diseases. It retains moisture in droughty times and drains well when conditions are wet. It sequesters carbon, nitrogen, and other nutrients that otherwise pollute our water and contaminate the atmosphere. Ultimately, our lives depend on it."

While industrial farmers feed plants chemical fertilizers to stimulate plant growth, organic farmers feed the soil. They apply compost made from decaying organic matter and manure, a valuable fertilizer, to build humus, which is vital to create good soil structure and enhance biological activity. Organic farmers plant cover crops and green manures, such as alfalfa and clover, to prevent soil erosion, reduce weeds, and provide nitrogen, a vital nutrient.

A handful of fertile soil may appear lifeless. In reality it teems with life, with billions of microorganisms, including bacteria, fungi, and algae, working in complex, cyclical interactions. Such biological activity creates nutrients to support plant growth.

One of the most important soil-building techniques used by organic farmers is crop rotation, which involves planting a succession of different crops on the same land year after year. Planting crops such as grasses adds vital nutrients back to the soil. In addition, crop rotation breaks insect and disease life cycles and suppresses weeds.

Many conventional farmers follow a two-year rotation, planting corn one year and soybeans the next. This requires heavy doses of fertilizers and pesticides and causes soil erosion. David Vetter follows a nine-year rotation that includes three years of grasses and legumes to enrich the soil. "We aim to preserve, conserve, and improve the soil's natural ability to produce," he says.

LIMITING PESTS AND WEEDS WITHOUT CHEMICALS

The National Organic Standards Board's definition of organic further states that organic "is based on minimal use of off-farm inputs and on management practices that restore, maintain and enhance ecological harmony."

Organic farmers, such as David Vetter, don't use "off-farm inputs," for example, toxic pesticides, to kill weeds and insects. Instead, they work with nature, creating conditions to attract predatory birds and insects, including ladybugs, lacewings, spiders, and wasps, to limit pests.

Other methods to eliminate weeds are a shallow stirring of surface soil cultivation to cut off and root them out; adding mulch, such as straw or wood chips to suppress their growth; increasing crop density to crowd them; and burning them using propane flame torches.

GREATER DIVERSITY

Industrial farming relies heavily on crop monocultures, plantings of a single crop such as corn, soybeans, or wheat, on hundreds or thousands of acres. Monocultures are vulnerable to pests and disease, require large amounts of chemical pesticides and fertilizers to sustain them, and cause soils to erode.

Organic farms are more diverse. David Vetter grows corn, popcorn, soybeans, barley, grasses, such as alfalfa and clover, and legumes. He also raises cattle on the grasses and sells them as grass-fed beef. Such diversity provides more ways to protect the crops from pests and drought and reduces financial risk that can result from a crop failure.

The advantages of crop diversity were dramatically demonstrated in China in 2000. Researchers discovered that growing two rice varieties instead of one monoculture greatly reduced the incidence of rice blast, the most damaging rice disease. The simple change increased rice yields significantly and allowed farmers to abandon the use of chemical fungicides that had been used to fight the disease.

ACCENTUATING THE POSITIVE

Eliot Coleman, a recognized expert on organic farming and author of *The New Organic Gardener,* views pests and disease not as a problem, but as an indicator that plants are weak and stressed. He says killing pests treats the symptom when the solution lies in strengthening the plant. Coleman writes, "The published research and the experience of organic growers around the world demonstrate clearly that when we accentuate the positive, we simultaneously eliminate the negative."

Coleman suggests this may also be the key to human health. "If we have followed this positive approach to plant health and have optimized all factors of the plant's growing conditions in order to turn out a plant of the highest biological quality, will the consumption of that plant be a factor in optimizing our nutrition and subsequent well-being?"

FEED THE WORLD?

Critics say organic agriculture cannot produce the high crop yields needed to feed an expanding world population. Not true. Research shows organic production matches or exceeds that of industrial agriculture. A study published in *Nature* compared conventional and organic apple production in Washington over a six-year period and found that the organic system produced better soil quality, comparable yields to conventional, higher profits, greater energy efficiency, and firmer, better-tasting apples. A long-term study at the University of California at Davis found that yields of organic tomato, safflower, corn, and beans equaled and, in some cases, exceeded conventional varieties. The Rodale Institute has compared yields of organic and conventional corn and soybeans for more than twenty years. "In our studies, yields in organic meet or exceed conventional yields," says Paul Hepperly, Rodale research and training manager.

GMO THREAT

Organic farming standards prohibit the use of genetically modified organisms (GMOs) or crops, seeing them as a short-term, shortsighted "fix" for industrial agriculture's problems and as a major threat to their crops, soil biology, the environment, and human health.

David Vetter lost money as a result of the incursion of GM crops on his farm. GM transgenes had contaminated his organic corn through wind-borne pollen from neighboring GM corn. His corn tested positive for GM material for several years, though at very low levels—0.1 percent—but enough to cost Vetter a customer.

As a result, the normally soft-spoken Vetter has become an outspoken critic of genetically modified crops not only because of their threat to his livelihood but also because of their risks to human health and the environment. When asked what the best solution is to the threat of GM crops to organic, he says simply, "a ban on GMOs."

GREATER OPPORTUNITIES FOR FAMILY FARMS

Organic agriculture provides greater income possibilities to small- and medium-size farms. Industrial agriculture pushes small farms to become larger and larger, which forces many farmers to either sell their small farms or find alternatives. Organic provides an excellent alternative because farmers can earn premium prices growing crops that have a high demand. The McCracken family discussed in Chapter 2 converted their small Iowa farm to organic for this reason.

David Vetter supports organic farmers in his area by purchasing their grains at fair prices and processing them in his Grain Place Foods facility. In addition, Grain Place Foods employs people from the local community, including pensioners and stay-at-home mothers who otherwise may not be able to find work.

Keeping family farmers in business and providing employment to people in small rural towns helps to sustain such communities, which are disappearing in America.

BIG PICTURE

Organic farmers view their work as part of a larger ecosystem, encompassing soil, plants, animals, biodiversity, natural resources, human beings, and communities. Their practices aim to protect, preserve, and sustain all these areas. Organic farmers recycle wastes on the farm and use no toxic chemicals and so protect public health and water supplies. They treat animals humanely with organic feed, access to outdoors, adequate sanitation, and no use of hormones or antibiotics. Organic farmers aim to preserve and increase wildlife habitats, such as wetlands. They use natural resources wisely. Research by the Rodale Institute has found that organic farming systems require 37 percent less fossil fuels than industrial agriculture.

The soil on David Vetter's farm developed under prairie grasses for thousands of years. He sustains that connection by planting ample grasses as part of his crop rotations, believing these will naturally enrich the native soil. In this way, Vetter hopes to "look at the impact 100 years ahead." With a smile he adds, "Wes Jackson [sustainable agriculture expert] says that's not long enough."

LONG-TERM VIEW

Today, David Vetter says he doesn't mind conventional farmers laughing at him. "Someone has to keep the coffee shop conversation interesting, it might as well be us," he says laughing.

Vetter's commitment to the long-term helped him outlast some of his critics. He remembers overhearing three farmers about twenty years ago talking about him, saying, "He won't last two or three years." Since then, all three of those farmers have gone out of business.

When asked what is needed to succeed as an organic farmer, Vetter says simply, "You have to have the commitment here," pointing to his heart.

Chapter 4

CERTIFIED ORGANIC

For a food to be labeled "organic," it must be certified as having been produced according to strict standards established by the U.S. Department of Agriculture's National Organic Program (NOP). Certified organic foods feature the green and white "USDA Organic" seal.

NEED FOR CERTIFICATION

Certification of organic foods began in the 1970s when organizations, such as California Certified Organic Farmers and the Northeast Organic Farming Association, saw the need to establish standards for producing and labeling organic foods. Farmers and food manufacturers that followed the standards would be "certified organic," which would enhance the credibility of their product and assure consumers of the product's quality.

As the organic food movement grew, more organic certification organizations were formed nationwide. The problem was that each certifier had its own standards and the term "organic" had no consistent meaning from state to state or from certifier to certifier, creating confusion. In addition, some food producers falsely promoted their products as organic when they weren't certified, which angered organic farmers and food companies who adhered to the rules.

NATIONAL ORGANIC PROGRAM

Leaders of the organic food movement saw the need to create consistent, uniform rules to apply nationwide. In the 1980s, they lobbied the government to create national organic rules. While most industries try to avoid government regulations, the organic industry asked for them. In 1990, Congress, led by Vermont Senator Patrick Leahy, passed the Organic Foods Production Act, which mandated rules for the production, handling, and marketing of organic foods. In 1992, the National Organic Standards Board, made up of farmers, retailers, environmentalists, and food manufacturers, was created to establish the rules.

As can happen when the government gets involved, developing the rules was a long and difficult process. In 1997, the USDA issued proposed rules allowing the use of irradiation, sewer sludge, and genetic engineering in organic foods. Outraged consumers flooded the USDA with 275,000 letters and e-mails protesting the proposals. The agriculture secretary at the time, Dan Glickman, said that the angry response was "so full-throated that I think it was choking me on occasion." As a result of the outcry, the USDA prohibited the controversial practices in organic foods.

"INTEGRITY AND AUTHENTICITY"

The NOP finally became law on October 21, 2002, and foods certified organic could display the green and white "USDA Organic" seal. The USDA accredited the original certification organizations, as well as new ones, state agencies, and international certifiers to certify organic foods according to the NOP. More than seventy certifiers worldwide are now accredited. Farmers and food manufacturers wanting to label their products organic must be certified by one of these firms.

The NOP represented a significant milestone for the United States organic movement. The law's passage enhanced its credibility, and fueled an even greater demand for organic food. Katherine DiMatteo, then executive director of the Organic Trade Association, said the NOP satisfied consumers' demand for one organic label. "They want to trust the integrity and authenticity of the organic claim," she said.

Not everyone is happy with the NOP. Many believe it is designed to help large farms and food manufacturers enter the organic market. Owners of small organic farms, in particular, feel left out. "A lot of small, regional farms can't afford the cost of certification," says Anthony Rodale, vice chairman of the Rodale Institute, which conducts organic farming research. "We really need some recognition for these farms so they can participate and be a part of a larger community."

ORGANIC RULES

The NOP rules formalize the ideals and practices of organic food production described in Chapter 3. In general, natural substances are allowed in organic production while synthetic substances are prohibited. As discussed earlier, the NOP prohibits the use of genetic engineering, irradiation, and sewage sludge. Other prohibited substances include synthetic insecticides, herbicides, fungicides, and fertilizers, as well as antibiotics and growth hormones in organic dairy, meat, and poultry.

Other NOP rules include the following:

- Farmland must be clear of prohibited substances, such as pesticides, for at least three years in order to be certified organic.

- Farmers must regularly rotate crops to maintain soil health.

- Farmers must use organically grown seeds, annual seedlings, and planting stock when commercially available.

- Farm animals must have sanitary housing, freedom of movement, and access to outdoors.

- Animals used to produce organic dairy, meat, and poultry must be fed 100 percent organic feed.

Critics say that organic farming's use of animal manure as fertilizer increases the risk that harmful bacteria may contaminate food produced in soil where it is used. However, the NOP recommends that farmers compost manure before use. Further, the NOP prohibits farmers from using raw manure unless it is incorporated into the soil 90 to 120 days prior to harvest of food crops for human consumption.

BEHIND THE ORGANIC LABEL: LUNDBERG FAMILY FARMS

While consumers see the organic label on foods, they don't see the time, effort, and expense that farmers and food manufacturers invest to certify their products as organic, from "farm to fork."

At Lundberg Family Farms, an organic rice grower and processor in Richvale, California, maintaining the organic certification is not an easy task. Lundberg's rice-farming operation encompasses 10,000 acres, which includes two Lundberg family-owned farms and twenty-three other family farms that grow rice for the Lundbergs. There are rice storage facilities and a manufacturing plant where Lundberg's organic rice products, including rice cakes, hot cereals, rice beverages, pasta, and syrup are made. Everything at Lundberg's, from the farm to finished food products, must be certified organic.

Sustainable farming is a four-generation-and-counting family tradition for the Lundbergs, starting in 1937 when Albert and Francis Lundberg and their four sons moved from Nebraska to the northern Sacramento Valley to escape the dust bowl disaster. Albert Lundberg brought with him sustainable farming practices and adapted them to growing rice. In the early 1960s his sons, Eldon, Wendell, Harlan, and Homer, established the family business, which since has grown to be one of the largest producers of organic rice in the world.

At Lundberg's, organic certification begins on the farms themselves. Farmers must plant organic seed and establish buffer zones to protect their rice from cross-pollination from neighboring rice fields. They must rotate cover crops to enrich the soil. Unlike conventional rice farmers, organic farmers don't burn rice straw after harvest. Instead, they let it decompose in the fields to nourish the soil and provide feed for migrating waterfowl. Lundberg's farmers also utilize water conserving irrigation practices.

Organic certification requires great attention to detail. Farmers must keep extensive records of their fields, the crops grown, inputs, seed purchases, compost practices, crop rotations, and pest and weed management methods, amongst other criteria.

In their storage and manufacturing facilities, the Lundbergs must prove that every step, from delivery and storage of rice to packaging of rice products, complies with NOP rules. They must avoid using prohibited substances and segregate organic rice products from their nonorganic products. They must provide detailed descriptions of products and ingredients used to make them. They must compile lists of all materials and equipment, pest controls, and cleaning products and procedures used. Product labels must follow NOP rules to the letter.

Organic inspectors conduct annual inspections of Lundberg's farms and facilities. They review records to ensure foods can be traced back through every stage of production. "Sometimes organic inspectors will pick a product and ask to see the audit trail tracing it back to the farmer's field," says Bryce Lundberg, director of organic certification at Lundberg Family Farms and third-generation family farmer.

Such "traceability" is increasingly important because of food scares, such as mad cow disease. Traceability enhances food security by allowing government and industry to trace the source of a food-borne illness. It also provides information to consumers about the origins of the foods they buy. With its extensive record keeping, organic certification has built-in traceability.

Organic certification provides the "proof in the pudding," says Lundberg, and assures consumers that a food product is produced to the highest quality standards. "Consumers want to know that a product is certified," he says. "It adds credibility to the claim that it was grown and produced organically."

UNDERSTANDING THE ORGANIC LABEL

Consumers can identify certified organic foods by the green and white "USDA Organic" label or by the statement "certified organic" along with the name of the organic certifier. The label is usually prominently displayed on the product or the package's main panel.

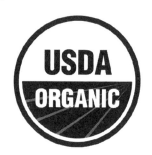

Certified organic foods are labeled according to the percentage of organic content found in the food. There are four categories of labels, but only the first two can display the "USDA Organic" Seal:

Figure 4.1.
USDA Organic Seal
of Approval

1. **"100% Organic."** These products contain only certified organic content. Examples are fruits and vegetables and other all-organic products such as milk, orange juice, cheese, eggs, chicken, and beef. In addition, some packaged foods may contain all organic content. *All products in this category may display the "USDA Organic" seal.*

2. **"Organic."** Products in this category must contain at least 95 percent certified organic content, excluding water and salt. Up to 5 percent of a product's ingredients may be nonorganic, but these ingredients must be approved under NOP rules. For example, some organic fruit jam products contain non-organic citric acid, a preservative, and pectin, a jelling agent. A wide range of foods feature this label, including baby foods, canned soups, cereals, cookies, frozen

vegetables, fruit jams, salad dressings, soymilk, and yogurt. *All products in this category may display the "USDA Organic" seal.*

3. **"Made With Organic."** Products in this category must contain at least 70 percent organic content. A product's main panel features the organic ingredients and may include up to three specific ingredients, for example, "Made With Organic Wheat, Corn, and Rice." Many packaged foods fall into this category, including cereals, cookies, corn chips, crackers, frozen foods, and yogurt.

4. **"Less than 70% Organic."** Products that contain less than 70 percent organic content may only list the organic content on the product label's ingredient list; it cannot be displayed on the product's main panel. For example, a product's ingredient list may contain "organic wheat" or "organic soybeans." Foods in this category include cookies, cereals, and baby foods.

Note: Not all food products that fit the criteria for "organic" will have the "USDA Organic" seal. Use of the USDA seal by food companies is voluntary, and some choose not to use it, but their products are still organic.

Lundberg Family Farms displays the USDA seal on its products. "We believe there is an acceptance by consumers that the USDA seal adds credibility," says Bryce Lundberg. "It adds to the claims of the producers."

INTERNATIONAL CERTIFICATION

Organic certification is a global endeavor. According to the International Federation of Organic Agriculture Movements (IFOAM), there are about 130 nations producing certified organic foods today. As well, more than 360 organizations in fifty-seven countries provide organic certification services. In addition, several nations, including those in the European Union, Argentina, Australia, Japan, and New Zealand, have established their own national organic standards. Others, such as Canada, are in the process of doing so.

Chapter 5

ORGANIC
LEGACY

*Organics is not a fad. It has been a long-established practice—
much more firmly grounded than the current chemical flair.
Present agricultural practices are leading us downhill.*

—J.I. Rodale, founder of Rodale, Inc., and publisher of
Organic Gardening and Farming, writing in 1954

It is clear that agriculture in general is going in the wrong direction.

—Anthony Rodale, vice chairman, the Rodale Institute,
writing in 2003

The entire philosophy behind organic foods may be best expressed by the few words on the sign that greets visitors to the Rodale Institute in Kutztown, Pennsylvania: "Healthy Soil, Healthy Food, Healthy People." This simple, time-honored formula has been tested, refined, and proven at the Rodale Institute for the past fifty years.

Located in a valley amidst the fertile rolling hills of eastern Pennsylvania, the Rodale Institute occupies a significant place in the past and future of organic food. The name Rodale has become synonymous with organic food through publications such as *Organic Gardening* and *Prevention* and pioneering research on organic farming. For three generations, the Rodale family has championed organic food, while researching and educating people about its benefits to soil, plant life, human health, and the environment. Each stage in the growth of the organic movement parallels the vision and work of each successive generation of Rodales.

ORGANIC PIONEERS

The roots of modern organic farming go back to the early 1900s, arising as a backlash against agriculture's increasing use of synthetic fertilizers. An early pioneer, Englishman Sir Albert Howard, studied organic farming methods practiced by peasant farmers of India and became convinced that the key to producing healthy food crops was to enhance the living organic or "humus" complex of the soil. Howard wrote, "The maintenance of the fertility of the soil is the first condition of any permanent system of agriculture." As a result of the work of Howard and other early organic pioneers, such as German scholar Rudolf Steiner, the humus farming movement grew throughout Europe from the 1920s to the 1950s.

Howard's writings greatly influenced J. I. Rodale, a magazine publisher from Emmaus, Pennsylvania. In 1940, Rodale purchased a sixty-acre farm near Emmaus to apply the humus farming methods. Encouraged by the farm's success, Rodale wrote and spoke out against chemical-intensive agriculture that began to dominate farming in the United States. Like Howard and other organic pioneers, he believed the key to human health was eating plants grown in healthy soil. He helped popularize the term "organic" and published the first magazine on organics, *Organic Gardening and Farming*.

In 1947, J. I. Rodale established the Soil and Health Foundation, whose mission was to "conduct, engage, foster, and encourage scientific research and study, teaching, training, informing and educating the public on and concerning the soil, food, and the health of people and their relationship to each other."

J. I. Rodale and fellow American organic pioneers, such as Paul Keene, founder of Walnut Acres Farm, faced hostile critics. A 1952 *Reader's Digest* article titled "Organic Agriculture—Bunk" blasted the new methods, which seemed odd compared to the new industrial agriculture with its "safe" chemical weapons that promised to eradicate disease and pests once and for all.

Silent Spring, Rachel Carson's landmark 1962 book that detailed hazards of agricultural chemicals, confirmed J. I. Rodale's beliefs and spurred an interest in organic food through the next decade. In 1971, a cover story in the *New York Times Magazine* hailed J. I. Rodale as "Guru of the Organic Food Cult."

PROVING THE VIABILITY OF ORGANIC

After J. I. Rodale's death in 1971, his son, Robert, continued and expanded his father's work. He became chairman of the burgeoning publishing business, Rodale, Inc. In 1972, Robert Rodale purchased a

330-acre farm in nearby Kutztown, establishing what is now the Rodale Institute. Robert Rodale aimed to prove the viability of what he called "regenerative agriculture."

"My father was ridiculed by researchers and government people," says Anthony Rodale, Robert's son and institute vice chairman. "They said, 'Organic farming is cute, but can it work on a large scale and be economically viable?'"

The Rodale Institute's research farm lies in a dale, or valley, with farmland stretching in all directions on the hilly terrain. It is an idyllic scene one imagines of rural America. An old one-room schoolhouse serves as the institute's welcome center and bookstore. Two apple orchards near the schoolhouse contain 900 trees bearing more than forty different apple varieties. A creek runs through the middle of the property. A large white clapboard farmhouse and the building behind it serve as offices for the institute's fifty employees. A self-guided tour around the farm helps visitors learn principles of organic farming through educational signposts along the path. Fertile organic fields are planted with grains, such as corn, oats, rye, soybeans, and wheat, as well as cover crops to build soil fertility. A three-acre plot is planted with vegetables for a local community-supported agriculture program.

"Institute" conjures images of academic buildings with researchers conducting laboratory experiments. The Rodale Institute's activities focus on the fields, conducting "living," long-term experiments to uncover the benefits of organic farming.

BOB RODALE'S VISION

"This is the crown jewel of the farm," says David Ward, institute vice president, as he walks to a twelve-acre field at the far edge of the farm. Ward refers to one of the living experiments, the farming systems trial, a long-term direct comparison of organic and conventional/chemical farming methods.

"This was a vision of Bob Rodale. It's the only one of its kind in the world," says Ward. Robert Rodale established the farming systems trial in 1981 to prove that organic farming was a viable alternative to conventional farming.

The field is divided into long, straight rows of corn, soybeans, and cover crops in various stages of growth and harvest. Three approaches are compared side-by-side. One is a conventional farming system using chemical fertilizers and pesticides. The other two are organic, one using animal manure to build soil fertility, the third using "green" manures, such as alfalfa. Corn and soybeans are grown in all three systems to model the dominant crop production system practiced in the United States.

After nearly twenty-five years, the trial has demonstrated the unique benefits of organic farming. "We have lots of data on how the systems perform," says Ward.

The trial shows that organic crops yield as much and sometimes more than conventional. In some cases, conventional corn grew faster at first, but organic corn plants ended up taller with longer cobs, 12 inches to 9 inches for conventional, says Ward. There are other differences. Organic crops use energy and water resources more efficiently, improve soil quality, and boost soil microbial activity. The organic soil looks noticeably blacker and more fertile. Organic crops demonstrate a striking environmental benefit: They absorb and retain carbon at significant levels, which may aid in reducing the impact of global warming. In addition, organic systems compete financially with conventional systems.

Published research is starting to document the benefits of organic farming discovered through the farming systems trial. A 2005 study published in *Bioscience* found that organic farming produces the same yields of corn and soybeans as does conventional farming but uses 30 percent less energy, less water, and no pesticides. Study lead author David Pimentel, a Cornell University professor of ecology and agriculture, said that organic methods also conserve more water in the soil, produce less erosion, maintain soil quality, and conserve more biological resources than conventional farming.

The farming systems trial is ongoing. "It's a living experiment. It doesn't have an end to it," says John Haberern, institute president. "It's always moving toward opening new frontiers of science, which will have long-term positive effects on human and environmental health." As Anthony Rodale says, "We will never have a full and complete understanding of the potential of organic."

The farming systems trial is one of many research projects conducted by the Rodale Institute. A study funded by the Pennsylvania Department of Environmental Protection found that compost provides optimum nutrient levels for crop growth while minimizing pollution of ground and surface water. A major food company is funding a study hoping to prove that organic foods are more nutritious than conventional; the company aims to state such a claim on its food labels. Another study will compare the nutritional value of organic, conventional, and genetically engineered feed on animals.

GOVERNMENT RECOGNITION

Robert Rodale continued pursuing his vision for organic until his death in 1990. In the mid-1980s, he and other organic proponents lobbied the government to recognize organic agriculture, leading to the creation of the Low Input Sustainable Agriculture program, which is now the Sustainable Agriculture Research and Education program (SARE), within the U.S. Department of Agriculture.

During those years, the American organic food movement continued to grow. A 1989 report by the National Resources Defense Council showing cancer risks posed by Alar, a common pesticide sprayed on apples, fueled sales of organic foods. By 1990 organic food sales reached more than $1 billion. That year, U.S. Congress passed the Organic Foods Production Act to establish consistent standards for producing organic food (see Chapter 4).

The same year, Robert Rodale was killed in a car accident while visiting Russia to establish *Novii Fermer,* a Russian magazine devoted to sustainable agriculture.

THIRD GENERATION VISION

J. I. and Robert Rodale have passed on, but their legacies—Rodale, Inc., the largest independent book publisher in the United States, and the Rodale Institute—continue to educate people about healthy food. "They educated and inspired two generations of farmers, researchers, and the public for nearly fifty years," says Anthony Rodale.

Anthony continues the work started by his grandfather and father while pursuing his own vision. "The issues facing each generation are different, but the overall goal of changing the way to grow and eat food has never changed," he says.

While his father and grandfather aimed to establish organic's credibility, Anthony Rodale wants to go further. He states, "My generation represents the 'adoption' phase, where we continue to research, educate, and spread the organic message to the mainstream."

NEWFARM.ORG

A key medium for spreading the organic message is *New Farm* (www.newfarm.org), which began as a magazine in 1979 and was reinvented as an online resource in 2002. *New Farm* provides resources and information about organic farming and food, aiming to create an online organic farming community.

One of the Rodale Institute's oldest buildings houses the institute's newest Internet technologies. A big white barn dating back to 1819 was converted to office space for *New Farm*. Stepping inside, a narrow corridor leads to small offices where *New Farm* editors write articles that provide "farmer-to-farmer know-how."

New Farm serves as a global resource for organic farmers where they can learn, share information, and see how much they can earn for crops. There is even a separate *New Farm Japan* site serving that nation's organic farmers.

Anthony Rodale wants to expand *New Farm*'s scope beyond farmers. "One of our biggest goals is to connect with the public through *New Farm*," he says. A step in that direction is Kidsregen.org, a web-based outreach program developed by Anthony's wife, Florence, that aims to "empower children to make healthy choices for the environment, and for themselves."

"WE DON'T HAVE TIME"

Anthony Rodale set a goal of 100,000 certified organic farmers in the United States by 2013, an ambitious vision considering there are now about 15,000. He says achieving that number will require help from the government, something that has been lacking to date. "The government treats organic as a young child when it could be a viable competitive choice for American farmers," he says.

Anthony Rodale's vision for organic extends beyond the United States. He sees the Rodale Institute as a worldwide organization. "One of the most important things I learned from my father and grandfather was that organic was a universal idea and that people worldwide understand it," he says. The Rodale Institute has launched international programs to foster regenerative agriculture in Senegal, Guatemala, and Russia. The Institute also has a partnership with a Japanese organization named Shinji Shumeikai, which includes spiritual leaders, farmers, and consumers.

Anthony Rodale feels a sense of urgency about the need for organic, regenerative agriculture worldwide. "We don't have time. The public is facing health and environmental problems," he says, pointing to the mounting evidence of negative effects caused by industrial agriculture. He also sees threats from increasing domination over food by agribusiness giants driven by profits at the expense of human health and the environment. "We need to think about health in a long-term point of view rather than greed and profit in short-term," he says.

SIMPLE FORMULA

Today, thanks to the work of the Rodale family and countless other organic heroes, the organic food movement is growing steadily, attracting more consumers, prospering financially, and achieving scientific credibility and government recognition. More important, organic is creating sustainable agriculture for future generations. It's all based on a simple Rodale formula: healthy soil, healthy food, and healthy people.

Chapter 6

HEALTHIER
BY NATURE

One day after spraying his fields with pesticides, Klaas Martens
tried folding the sprayer to put it away but discovered that he
couldn't move his right arm. It was paralyzed.

"It was scary," says his wife, Mary-Howell, recalling the incident.

Martens's instant paralysis was caused by exposure to the toxic
pesticides he sprayed on the couple's 1,300-acre farm in Penn Yan,
New York.

He later regained movement in the arm thanks to chiropractic treat-
ments, but the paralysis was the latest in a series of health problems
caused by pesticide exposure. There were also headaches and nausea.

Martens dreaded spraying. "I knew I would feel rotten for a month
after," he says.

He suffered despite taking precautions. While spraying, Martens
wore a white, head-to-toe Tyvek suit with green plastic gloves.

Mary-Howell hated to see her husband suffer. Years later, she
wrote, "We wanted to believe that it [his sickness] was due to 'just a
germ' since he had been working such long hours, but we knew better.
My husband was slowly being poisoned."

PESTICIDE HEALTH HAZARDS

Klaas Martens's experience highlights the biggest health hazard of
industrial agriculture: pesticide exposure. Pesticides are extremely toxic substances, used to kill insects, weeds, and plant diseases, such as
fungi. Just a few drops ingested can kill an average person. This fact is
particularly disturbing considering that *2 billion pounds* of chemical
pesticides are used in the United States each year, with most of that
doused on farmland.

As a result of such widespread use, pesticide residues are every-
where—in our air, soil, water, food, and bodies. A 2004 report by the
Pesticide Action Network (PAN) states that blood and urine analyses

of 9,282 individuals by the U.S. Centers for Disease Control and Prevention (CDC) found that *every* person contained an average of thirteen to twenty-three pesticide residues in their bodies. According to tests conducted by the U.S. Department of Agriculture, about 80 percent of 21,807 samples of conventionally grown fresh fruits contained one or more pesticide residues. Some fruits and vegetables were found to contain up to 4.2 different residues.

Pesticide exposure is linked to cancer, brain damage, weakened immunity, endocrine system disruptions, and reproductive problems. While it is difficult to definitively prove a direct causal link between pesticide exposure and a particular illness or disease, scientists have concluded that pesticide exposure increases the likelihood that certain health problems will occur or lead to serious illness. Evidence of health problems linked to pesticide exposure is mounting:

- Researchers at the University of Missouri, Columbia found that men living in agricultural areas had sperm counts as much as 40 percent lower than men living in major cities, such as New York and Los Angeles. Runoff from farm chemicals is the suspected cause.

- University of Rochester researchers found that maneb, a fungicide commonly used in farming, damages brain cells, paving the way for Parkinson's disease.

- A University of Wisconsin study found that combinations of commonly used agricultural pesticides and fertilizers, in concentrations similar to those found in groundwater, can significantly influence the immune and endocrine systems as well as neurological health. The study suggested that current methods used by the Environmental Protection Agency (EPA) and others for studying the toxic effects of low-levels of pesticides may be flawed.

Farm workers, such as Klaas Martens, are especially at risk for pesticide-related illnesses. The EPA estimates there are 10,000 to 20,000 physician-diagnosed pesticide illnesses and injuries per year related to farm work.

"THOUSANDS UPON THOUSANDS OF DEATHS"

Pesticides pose an especially great risk to children. A growing body of scientific research links prenatal pesticide exposure, as well as exposure during the first years of a child's life, to health problems such as low birth weight, birth defects, abnormal neurological development, and reproductive problems.

"Pesticides in children is a big deal," says Alan Greene, M.D., a pediatrician and faculty member at Stanford University School of Medicine. According to Greene, pesticides are directly responsible for premature births, which is the leading cause of death in babies, stunted brain growth, and learning disabilities.

He cites a CDC study analyzing DDT pesticide levels in blood samples taken from 44,000 pregnant women between 1959 and 1966. The study found a 50 percent increase in premature births among women who had small levels of DDT in their blood and a 300 percent increase among women who had high levels. Based on the study, Greene says DDT was "responsible for thousands upon thousands of deaths."

Greene says pesticides used today are even more toxic and are directly linked to prematurity, as well as other health problems, including cancer and asthma. "Far more Americans have been killed by the chemicals we put on our food than by the September 11 terrorist attacks and the war in Iraq," he says.

PROTECTION FROM PESTICIDES

In 1991, Klaas and Mary-Howell Martens reached a crossroads. The Martens farmed "conventionally" using pesticides because they saw no alternative. But, according to Mary, they "hated what it might be doing to us, our family, our land, and our environment."

Later that year, they read a classified ad in a farm newspaper looking for organic wheat. Klaas called, and the Martens decided to try organic farming.

By switching to organic, the Martens stopped using pesticides, and by doing so, dramatically reduced their health risks associated with pesticides.

Similarly, consumers who eat organic foods reduce their exposure to health-damaging pesticides. A 2002 study conducted by the Organic Materials Review Institute and Consumers Union, publisher of *Consumer Reports* magazine, confirmed that organic foods contain significantly fewer pesticides than conventionally produced foods. Researchers analyzed test data from more than 94,000 organic and non-organic food samples of about twenty different crops tested over nearly a decade. Results showed that 73 percent of conventionally grown produce had at least one pesticide residue, while only 23 percent of organically grown samples contained residues. In California, pesticide residues were found in nearly a third of conventionally grown foods, compared to just 6.5 percent of organic samples.

A landmark 2002 study conducted by researchers at the University of Washington's School of Public Health and Community Medicine found that preschool children eating a diet of organic foods had six to nine times lower pesticide levels in their bodies than children eating conventional foods. The authors concluded, "Consumption of organic produce appears to provide a relatively simple means for parents to reduce their children's exposure to organophosphorus pesticides."

It is important to note that while organic food standards prohibit the use of pesticides, trace residues may be found on organic foods because pesticides are pervasive in the environment. Pesticides sprayed on fields can drift for many miles, contaminating organic crops, they may seep into water supplies used to irrigate organic crops, and they may remain active in soils long after being applied.

MORE ANTIOXIDANTS IN ORGANIC

In recent years, scientists have discovered the health benefits of antioxidants, vital nutrients found naturally in the human body and in fruits and vegetables. Antioxidants promote health by neutralizing free radicals, unstable molecules that damage healthy cells through a process called oxidation. In the same way that a car rusts, oxidation damages and kills healthy cells, which can speed the aging process and lead to health problems, such as heart disease, cancer, and weakened immunity.

Antioxidants scavenge free radicals and transform them into non-damaging compounds. This prevents cellular damage, which in turn slows aging, strengthens immunity, and decreases the risk of cancer and other health problems.

Common antioxidants include vitamins A, C, and E and compounds called carotenoids, such as beta-carotene, which gives fruits and vegetables deep, rich color. Lycopene, which is found in tomatoes, is considered to be another beneficial antioxidant. Deep-colored fruits and vegetables, such as blueberries, plums, strawberries, broccoli, and red cabbage, are rich in antioxidants.

A 2005 report by the Organic Center for Education and Prevention found that, on average, antioxidant levels were about 30 percent higher in organic food compared to conventional food grown under the same conditions. The report reviewed fifteen quantitative comparisons of antioxidant levels in organic versus conventional fruit and vegetables and found that organically grown produce had higher levels in thirteen out of fifteen cases.

ORGANIC IS TOUGHER

Kathleen Merrigan, Ph.D., director of the agriculture, food and environment program at Tufts University, suggests that higher antioxidant levels in organic foods may be due to the fact that organic crops must activate defense mechanisms to ward off pests and disease, while conventional crops, which rely on pesticides, don't. These plant protection mechanisms may stimulate production of antioxidants. "Organic crops have to be tough, and this may increase antioxidant capacity," she says.

Merrigan and other researchers at Tufts University are conducting research to identify how organic farming methods affect antioxidant levels in fruits and vegetables.

Other studies have found higher antioxidant levels in organic foods:

- The Danish Institute of Agricultural Sciences found that organic milk contains significantly more vitamin E, higher levels of carotenoids, and two-to-three times more beta-carotene than conventional milk.

- U.S. Department of Agriculture scientists found that organic ketchup contains more than 50 percent higher levels of lycopene than conventional brands. The average level in the organic brands was by far the highest—174.2 micrograms per gram of ketchup compared to 110.7 micrograms per gram in the major conventional brands.

- A study by food scientists at the University of California, Davis, and published in the *Journal of Agricultural and Food Chemistry*, found that organic corn had 52 percent more vitamin C than conventional corn. The study also found that organic marionberries, a type of blackberry, contain significantly higher levels of polyphenols, which are cancer-fighting antioxidants, than conventionally grown foods.

WHOLE IS GREATER THAN THE SUM OF THE PARTS

It makes sense that eating foods grown in fertile, healthy soil and produced without toxic chemicals would be more nutritious, and emerging research is proving this.

However, it is important to remember that organic is a food production *process* where the whole is greater than the sum of the parts. Craig Holdrege, director and senior researcher at the Nature Institute, says, "The idea that food contains individual nutrients needs to be expanded. We need to look at food and health as a process."

Holdrege says consumers buy organic because they want to support this life-sustaining process. They want food produced without chemical pesticides and genetic engineering. They want to know that it protects the environment. They want to know the food's origin, and that it supports family farms. The fact that organic is healthier, says Holdrege, "is bound to the system."

"MADE FARMING FUN AGAIN"

Those who live the organic process every day, farmers such as Klaas and Mary-Howell Martens, may appreciate its value the most. They made the transition from industrial to organic farming and never looked back. They see continuing improvement in soil quality with fewer weeds. They earn a good living, enjoy the independence, and can set their own destiny. Without the pesticides, Mary-Howell says, "The farm is a safe place."

The Martens say the organic process helps rebuild the farming community. "It creates an environment where a family can thrive and children will want to stay," says Mary-Howell. The Martens' sixteen-year-old son, Peter, farms his own 100 acres, which gives him a sense of accomplishment and pride, says Klaas.

Finally, the Martens simply enjoy organic farming. As Klaas says, "It's made farming fun again."

LOCAL ORGANIC:
RESTORING THE VITAL LINK

*Farmers markets are one of the saviors of the family farm. All those
barriers created by the conventional system are torn down. The consumer
sees it isn't just a commodity—it's a peach, or a carrot, or a cabbage.*

—David Mas Masumoto, peach grower and writer

Every Saturday morning from the end of April until the beginning of
November, Capital Square in the heart of Madison, Wisconsin,
transforms into a street festival teeming with thousands of people.
There are street musicians performing for small crowds, artists and
crafts people selling their creations, and nonprofit groups promoting
their causes.

But all those activities are secondary to the main event: the Dane
County Farmers Market. Held on the green, tree-lined grounds surrounding the spectacular Wisconsin state capital building, the farmers
market attracts huge crowds that come to buy Wisconsin-made foods,
many of them organic. People come to connect directly with the source
of their food: farmers. They come to learn how their food is grown or
made and to enjoy fresh, locally produced fruits, vegetables, meats,
cheeses, and other foods.

"It's a happening place on Saturday mornings, that's for sure," says
Larry Johnson, Dane County Farmers Market manager.

NUMBER OF FARMERS MARKETS INCREASED
111 PERCENT

Here in Madison, and in cities and towns throughout the United States,
an age-old tradition, the farmers market, is re-emerging. Spurred by
consumers' desire for local, fresh, and good-tasting food, farmers markets are booming nationwide. According to the U.S. Department of
Agriculture, the number of farmers markets increased from 1,755 in
1994 to 3,706 in 2004, a phenomenal growth of 111 percent.

In New York City, more than 250,000 people visit Greenmarket farmers markets held in thirty-three locations throughout the city. More than eighty farmers markets are held in Chicago and surrounding suburbs each week throughout the summer. Seattle's Pike Place Market, the nation's oldest farmers market, encompasses nine acres and attracts an estimated 9 million customers each year.

Farmers markets are springing up in small towns too, such as Fairfield in rural Iowa (population 10,000) and Collingswood in suburban New Jersey (population 15,000), where a farmers market is held in a police station parking lot every Saturday morning from spring through fall.

In an age of cookie cutter fast-food chains selling foods produced who knows where, and supermarkets selling row upon row of highly processed, nutritionally suspect foods that travel thousands of miles, more and more consumers want healthier organic alternatives produced by local farmers.

"ONE-ON-ONE CONTACT WITH FARMERS"

The Dane County Farmers Market is the largest "producer-only" farmers market in the United States. This means all products are grown or made by the vendors selling them, and all are produced in Wisconsin.

"A whole gamut of products are sold," says Johnson. Seasonal vegetables range from asparagus to zucchini. Fruits include apples, grapes, pears, plums, and strawberries. There are cheeses and fourteen different meats, ranging from the traditional—beef, pork, and poultry—to the unusual—ostrich, bison, and emu. There are breads, candies, fruit jams, honey, maple syrup, pasta, snacks, sprouts, flowers, and plants—300 products in all.

Many foods are organic, some are conventional, and others are in between. Some farmers sell organic products that aren't certified. "Some of the older farmers complain, 'I don't want the damn paperwork [required for certification],'" says Johnson.

Johnson says people like connecting with farmers. "They can ask the producer how they grew the food and what their growing techniques are," he says.

People come to the farmers market for many reasons. "The choice, freshness, variety, and one-on-one contact with farmers are all very important," says Johnson.

CSA: "FOOD WITH THE FARMER'S FACE ON IT"

One of the mainstay vendors at the Dane County Farmers Market is Harmony Valley Farms, an organic vegetable farm owned and operated by Richard de Wilde and his wife, Linda Halley. Harmony Valley produces organic vegetables on seventy acres of land in a picturesque, fertile valley amidst the hills of southwestern Wisconsin.

Harmony Valley Farms operates a community supported agriculture (CSA) program. In a CSA, subscribers pay a membership fee to a local farmer in return for weekly deliveries of fresh organic produce throughout the growing season. CSA establishes a mutually beneficial relationship between farmers and consumers. Farmers gain a ready market and fair compensation for their crops, while consumers receive fresh, locally grown organic foods at prices below retail. Money remains in the community, supporting small, family farms. "It's a practical way to earn income on the farm," says Halley.

The CSA concept was first developed in Japan during the 1960s. A group of women, concerned with the increasing use of pesticides, established direct relationships with farmers and consumers. The Japanese term for CSA, "teikei," means "food with the farmer's face on it."

CSA eliminates unnecessary links in the food chain to connect consumers directly to farmers. Consumers learn how food is produced, gain a greater appreciation for farmers' work, and even participate in the farming work. In addition, CSA saves energy because no long distance transportation costs are involved.

Like farmers markets, CSA programs are fast-growing in the United States, increasing from just two in 1986 to 1,700 in 2004. These CSA programs feed 340,000 families each week.

Harmony Valley's 450 CSA members receive boxes of organic produce each week from May through December, paying from $22.50 to $26.00 per box. Harvested vegetables are washed, boxed, and delivered to drop-off sites in Madison and other nearby towns.

Harmony Valley provides more than forty varieties of fruits and vegetables, many that are not sold in stores. These include broccoli romanesco, cipollini onions, gold beets, heirloom tomatoes, purple cauliflower, "sunchoke" Jerusalem artichokes, wild leeks, and yellow carrots. "Every year we try growing something new," says Halley.

What draws people to CSA? "People want fresh and local food," says Halley. "They are unhappy with the quality of food in grocery stores. They also like the fact that they are sustaining a farm."

"A LOT OF ENTHUSIASM FOR LOCALLY GROWN"

Buying locally produced organic foods at farmers markets and through CSA programs represents a significant trend within the larger organic food movement. In fact, many consumers prefer local over organic. A study by the Leopold Center for Sustainable Agriculture at Iowa State University found that consumers are more likely to purchase locally grown foods over organic foods produced in a distant region, even if the local foods were produced using some pesticides. The study found that the term "locally grown" commands a great deal of power and influence for consumers, and consumers better understand the meaning of "locally grown" than "certified organic." In addition, 20 percent of consumers said they were willing to pay 30 percent or more for food products that combine the attributes of locally grown with environmental and community stewardship.

An Ohio State University study found that 59 percent of consumers would pay 10 percent more to purchase locally produced foods. Study researcher Jeff Sharp, a rural sociologist with the Ohio State University Extension, says, "We're seeing quite a lot of enthusiasm among consumers for locally grown foods."

FRESHER, BETTER TASTE, ENVIRONMENTALLY FRIENDLY

Locally produced foods offer many advantages. They are fresher and taste better than fruits and vegetables sold in grocery stores, which can travel as long as fourteen days before reaching stores. While farmers produce local varieties for taste and quality, supermarket varieties are chosen for durability in shipping and long shelf life. Anyone who has grown garden vegetables knows there's no comparison between a just-picked, fresh tomato—deep red, juicy, and delicious—and the lifeless, hard tomatoes found in supermarkets.

Buying locally gives consumers a greater choice of produce, including rare heirloom varieties not sold in stores, such as those grown by Harmony Valley Farms. These unique fruits and vegetables have been grown and passed down for generations by families throughout the world. Heirloom varieties offer an incredible diversity. Seed Savers Exchange, based in Decorah, Iowa, collects and preserves 25,000 heirloom varieties of fruits and vegetables, including 5,500 different tomatoes, 1,000 lettuces, and 700 apple varieties. In light of this full spectrum of heirloom varieties, the produce selection at most supermarkets—the common beefsteak tomato, iceberg lettuce, and Red and Golden Delicious apples—appears dim by comparison.

Consumers receive higher quality at a better price buying directly from farmers. Harmony Valley's CSA members pay 10 to 15 percent less for vegetables than they would pay in supermarkets or natural food cooperatives.

There may even be health benefits to eating locally grown foods. People who eat honey collected by bees in their area often develop immunity to pollen in that region. Local fruits and vegetables picked and eaten at the height of ripeness not only taste better but are likely to be more nutritious as well.

Buying local conserves energy and protects the environment. Another study by the Leopold Center found that food sold in Iowa supermarkets travels an average of 1,546 miles from the farm to the retail shelf, while food produced and sold by local farmers travels an average of forty-five miles. The study also found that the conventional food system uses four to seventeen times more fuel and emits five to seventeen times more carbon dioxide greenhouse gases than the local and regional systems, depending on the system and truck type.

Nearly every state buys as much as 90 percent of its food from somewhere else, causing billions of dollars to leak from state economies each year. Buying local keeps money circulating within communities. Farmers who sell directly to consumers through farmers markets and CSA programs earn more money without a middleman.

Because locally produced foods tend to be organic or produced using sustainable farming methods, consumers are protected from pesticides, genetic engineering, and other practices that threaten human health and the environment.

In an age of terrorist fears, buying local helps ensure food safety. Jennifer Wilkins, a food and society policy fellow at Cornell University, points out that a terrorist attack on a food system based on local production, with complex networks of farmers and processors intertwined with local communities, would be nearly impossible. "Strengthening local food systems and supporting policies that shorten the distance between producers and consumers will reduce the points of vulnerability and make America truly food-secure," says Wilkins.

Local food systems could also prevent food shortages caused by natural disasters such as hurricanes, which are increasing in frequency and intensity as a result of global warming.

Finally, and perhaps most important, local food production reestablishes the vital link between farmers and consumers that has been severed by industrial agriculture. Consumers learn who produces their food, how they produce it, and gain a greater appreciation for farmers' efforts. In turn, farmers learn who their customers are and can adjust their production to meet their wishes. Linda Halley says her CSA members often request certain vegetable varieties. "Our members offer ideas, usually good ideas," she says.

LOCAL ORGANIC IN SCHOOLS, RESTAURANTS, AND SUPERMARKETS

Farmers markets and CSA are just two examples of the local organic trend. An increasing number of schools, colleges, and universities buy locally produced organic foods to serve to their students. This trend is discussed in Chapter 8.

Many restaurants now serve meals made with locally produced organic vegetables and ingredients. Alice Waters, owner of the award-winning Chez Panisse in Berkeley, California, has developed a network of local farmers and ranchers that supply her restaurant with fresh organic ingredients. Waters, a leading local/organic food advocate, also established the Edible Schoolyard to teach children how to grow, harvest, and prepare organic food. Rick Bayless, award-winning chef and owner of Fronterra Grill and Topolobampo Mexican restaurants in Chicago, uses local organic produce extensively and advocates their use in restaurants nationwide. In Atlantic City, New Jersey, chef Luke Palladino, who operates two Italian restaurants, contracts with a local organic farmer to produce organic greens, mushrooms, and other seasonal vegetables. The Farmers Diner in Quechee, Vermont, serves organic food produced by local farmers. Devotay in Iowa City, Iowa, offers "local food with a worldly flair."

Supermarket chains now offer local organic. In Michigan, more than 200 stores, including Kroger and Super Kmart, sell local fruits and vegetables as part of a "Select Michigan" campaign. In southwest Virginia, forty organic farmers joined together to create the Appalachian

Harvest organic network. The farmers grow and sell organic produce to 150 stores owned by supermarket chains, including Ukrops, White's, Food City, and Whole Foods Markets in Virginia, eastern Tennessee, and North Carolina. The produce contains the Appalachian Harvest logo featuring a sun rising over a green valley with the tagline, "Healthy Foods, Healthy Farms, Close to Home." In Lincoln, Nebraska, a group of disgruntled corn and soybean farmers opened their own grocery store to sell food grown and made by Nebraska family farmers.

"LINKING PEOPLE WITH FOOD THAT MATCHES THEIR VALUES"

One of the most ambitious local food initiatives is FamilyFarmed.org, which aims to link organic farmers in Illinois and nearby states with Chicago restaurants and supermarkets. Jim Slama, president of Sustain, launched FamilyFarmed.org to help local farmers access the market, which Slama describes as a "huge opportunity" for them. "There is a strong consumer base that wants organic and local," he says.

FamilyFarmed.org's website allows consumers to find local farmers and read profiles about them and their products. "This helps connect consumers with farmers," says Slama.

Twelve Chicago-area supermarket chains comprising 125 stores participate in FamilyFarmed.org and sell locally produced organic foods. Each product displays the FamilyFarmed.org logo and includes information about the producing farmer.

Slama cites benefits created by local food production, such as reduced transportation costs and less pollution, but says consumers benefit the most. "They receive fresher, safer, and more nutritious organic food," he says. "This is about linking people with food that matches their values."

"GET YOURSELF A FARMER"

In Iowa, Kamyar Enshayan, an adjunct professor of physics at the University of Northern Iowa, organized a successful Buy Fresh Buy Local campaign that began in one city and has spread throughout the state.

"The way food is produced is not working. The food economy is disconnected from the land around us," says Enshayan, pointing to the irony that Iowa supermarkets contain foods produced thousands of miles away, while surrounding fertile farmland produces only corn and soybeans, mainly for animal feed. "There is nothing locally produced in a grocery store," he says.

In 1998, Enshayan convinced a local hospital, restaurant, and university to buy locally produced food. All found that local food was fresher, tasted better, and cost less than food supplied from traditional, far away sources. Today twenty-three institutions participate in the project, purchasing $500,000 a year from local farmers.

Enshayan estimates that if people in his region purchased just 10 percent of their food from local sources, it would keep $40 million within the region.

One small restaurant, Rudy's Tacos, purchases 71 percent of its food from local farmers. Rudy's places small signs on each table featuring photos of local farmers with the words "Rudy's invests in local farms."

The Buy Fresh Buy Local campaign provides local farmers with markets, gives local institutions fresh, wholesome foods, and keeps money circulating within local communities.

Most important, consumers connect with and learn about the source of their food, local farmers. "We want to reshape the food system in a different way," Enshayan says. "The slogan of industrial food production is 'Just eat it'—and don't question how it was produced. We want to ask where it came from and create a different slogan, 'Get yourself a farmer.'"

Chapter 8

ORGANIC MAKES THE GRADE IN SCHOOLS AND COLLEGES

The garden has changed my life here at Yale. It is a place where I engage my hands and my heart, a place I shape life and watch it grow, a place where I never stop deeply appreciating the earth.

—Laura Hess, Yale University student who participates in the Sustainable Food Project that introduced organic, locally produced foods into the university's dining halls

The dining hall at Maharishi University of Management in Fairfield, Iowa, appears more like a mini-United Nations than a college cafeteria. With students from more than fifty countries, including Belarus, Brazil, China, Ethiopia, India, Malaysia, Nepal, Norway, Pakistan, and the Philippines, to name a few.

Then there is the food. Everything—from the zucchini in the stir-fry to the chocolate chips in the desserts—is organic. Most of the vegetables are grown on the university's farm, and are freshly picked, cooked, and served, often on the same day.

Students appreciate the organic emphasis. "I'm definitely happy with that," says Nicole Windenberger, an American student. "Eating organic helps to create a sustainable environment, and the food tastes a lot better."

Thousands of students, like Windenberger, at schools and colleges throughout the United States are discovering the value of organic and locally produced foods.

Organic is appearing on school menus for several reasons. Parents and administrators, concerned about increasing child obesity rates due to poor diets, want young students to eat healthier foods. Health- and environmentally conscious college students want nutritious, natural foods. Teachers want students to learn about how and where food is produced, while farmers see schools as new markets for their organic crops.

FARM TO SCHOOL

According to Anupami Joshi, director of the National Farm to School Program, 400 school districts in twenty-three states buy locally produced and organic foods. "The program is growing rapidly, especially in the last couple of years," she says.

Farm to School aims to encourage schools to buy locally produced foods, to establish gardens at schools, and to educate students about nutrition and how farmers produce their foods.

Education is especially important. "We want to link what is being offered to them in the cafeteria with what is offered to them in classroom," says Joshi. Farmers come to schools to speak with students, and schools organize tours of farms so students can see how food is produced. As a result, Joshi says, "Students understand that they should eat more fruits and vegetables and to eat locally to support local farmers." Getting children to appreciate healthy foods at a young age gives them a foundation for a healthier life.

While Farm to School emphasizes buying locally over organic, there is often little difference between the two. "Local is the higher priority, but when you buy from small farmers they are using sustainable methods," says Joshi.

Joshi says Farm to School creates a win-win situation for everyone involved. Children eat better foods, which makes parents happy, school districts improve education about the importance of local foods, and farmers gain new markets, which keeps them on the land for everyone's benefit.

WISCONSIN HOME GROWN LUNCH

A good example of a farm to school program is Wisconsin Homegrown Lunch, which provides organic meals to students in several Madison, Wisconsin, schools.

Project coordinator Doug Wubben says the project, which received funding from a USDA Sustainable Agriculture Research and Education grant, aims to make locally produced foods more accessible to people who cannot afford organic foods.

A major driving force for projects like Wisconsin Homegrown Lunch is a concern over child obesity. According to a 2000 survey by the Centers for Disease Control and Prevention, 15 percent of children and teens ages six to nineteen are overweight, triple the number from

1980. "The obesity crisis has created the climate to allow our project to get the attention it has," says Wubben. "We are positioning this as a solution."

Wisconsin Homegrown Lunch launched a pilot project in three elementary schools and one middle school. Eight organic farmers provide vegetables, including tomatoes, potatoes, onions, and broccoli, to the schools. In addition, the project developed a meal—a chicken and vegetable tortilla wrap with a sweet potato muffin and a local apple—that is served at all the district's schools.

There are challenges. Food service kitchens usually receive foods that are already packaged and processed, making the introduction of fresh, unprocessed vegetables difficult. "They need food in prepared form to put in their system," says Wubben. In addition, schools require food throughout the year, but some farmers can only provide produce during their growing seasons.

Wisconsin Homegrown Lunch's education activities include bringing farmers into classrooms to speak to children, giving children the opportunity to taste different fruits and vegetables, and taking them on farm tours. Children have also had the opportunity to take home seedling tomato plants and plant them in their yards to gain a direct experience of growing food. "We are trying to create a connection of where food comes from, and if children have more knowledge about that, they are more willing to eat it," says Wubben.

There are many other examples of organic in schools. The Seattle, Washington, school district adopted a policy banning junk food and introducing organic food in school cafeterias. Each of the fifteen schools in California's Santa Monica-Malibu School District provides a salad bar containing fruits and vegetables purchased at local farmers markets. Stonyfield Farms, a New Hampshire-based manufacturer of organic dairy products, introduced healthy vending machines, containing organic snacks, such as yogurt smoothies, fruit juices, soymilk, and energy bars, into schools in six states.

ORGANIC ON CAMPUS

College and university students are also eating organic foods. An estimated 200 colleges have farm to college programs, according to Kristen Markley, Farm to College program manager for the nonprofit Community Food Security Coalition.

College students often initiate organic food programs. "Students want healthier food with a lower environmental impact," says Markley. A survey by Y-Pulse, a market and media research firm, confirms this premise. Twenty-five percent of young adults ages eighteen to twenty-five said that eating organic was important to them.

In 2001, students at Yale University launched the Sustainable Food Project to introduce organic foods into the university's dining halls. The project received strong support from Alice Waters, chef of Chez Panisse restaurant in Berkeley, California, whose daughter was then a freshman at Yale.

Meals produced from local, organic foods were served in Yale's Berkeley College Dining Hall starting in 2003. The project has become so popular that the number of students eating at Berkeley has nearly doubled. Organic foods served include vegetables and dairy products, such as cabbage, eggplant, greens, milk, potatoes, winter squash, yogurt, and zucchini. As a result of the project's success, there are plans to serve organic milk, fruit, and grass-fed beef in other Yale dining halls.

There are other examples of colleges serving organic food:

- The University of Wisconsin's Housing Food Service serves organic apples, blue corn chips, beef, corn, and potatoes. All hamburgers are made from organic beef. Many of the foods come from local farmers. Organic soymilk and milk are sold in university convenience stores. The university's Center for Integrated Agricultural Systems organizes an all-organic meal each semester to help educate students about the value of organic.

- A student survey at Princeton University found that more than 70 percent would choose organic foods over conventional. In response, Princeton's Dining Services decided to purchase organic and locally produced foods whenever possible. In 2004, Princeton purchased 760 pounds of organic cereal, 2,900 pounds of organic salad mix, and 23,000 pounds of locally produced food.

- Students at Oberlin College in Ohio launched a campaign to introduce organic and local foods in 1999. Since 2002, all of the milk served in Oberlin's dining halls has been organic. The school spends as much as 5 percent of its food budget on locally produced foods. In addition, food waste is composted at the college's seventy-acre farm.

- Other colleges serving organic and local foods include Stanford, Brown, Colorado College, Pennsylvania College of Technology, University of Northern Iowa, and Middlebury College in Vermont, to name a few.

ORGANIC "TO THE NTH DEGREE"

As a result of its successful Sustainable Food Project, Yale sometimes receives calls from other universities wanting advice on introducing organic foods. But when Yale's food distributor needed advice on buying organic, it contacted Tom Siegel, food service director at Maharishi University of Management (MUM).

No college or university has made as strong a commitment to serving organic as MUM. According to Siegel, who organizes meals for 700 people a day, as much as 95 percent of the food served at the university is organic.

The impetus to serve only organic came from university administrators who were concerned about the potential hazards of genetically engineered foods and wanted to avoid serving them to students. "The best way to do that is to buy certified organic," says Siegel.

MUM is an accredited university that integrates traditional learning disciplines, such as arts, sciences, and business, into a unique "consciousness-based" approach involving regular practice of Transcendental Meditation (TM) and other technologies drawn from the age-old Vedic tradition of India. Such techniques aim to raise the consciousness of individuals to greater health, happiness, and success in life and the consciousness of the world to greater peace and harmony.

Siegel says students who attend MUM tend to be health and environmentally conscious and appreciate the organic emphasis. "They have greater goals of wanting to help the environment and raise world consciousness, and they want to eat organic food because it is better for their health," he says. MUM's educational approach attempts to raise world consciousness by raising the consciousness of individuals through the practice of TM and related techniques. This approach is said to be effective because all individuals are connected and interrelated at the basis of life, which is the "field" of consciousness.

Nicole Windenberger, a student in MUM's Sustainable Living program, says she has learned about the value of organic food attending the university. "A couple of years ago I wouldn't have appreciated it, but we get repeated exposure [to its importance] from our teachers," she says. Today, she says, "I can't eat non-organic fruit anymore because of the pesticide residues found on conventional fruit."

The fact that the food is produced locally is also important to Windenberger. "Local makes a big difference in terms of freshness and supporting the local economy," she says. "You find out who's growing your food. Many people don't know where their food comes from."

Everything served at MUM, including beans, breads, canned goods, cereals, dairy products, desserts, flavors, flours, fruit jams, fruits, grains, oils, pasta, potato chips, spices, sweeteners, and vegetables, is organic. "We're going to the nth degree," says Siegel.

The salad bar is filled with farm-fresh lettuce, daikon radishes, shredded beets and carrots, spinach, cucumbers, tofu, cottage cheese, yogurt, and five kinds of sprouts.

The only time MUM purchases non-organic food is when items, such as black olives, nut butters, and certain spices, are too expensive or are not available as organic.

Siegel says the price difference between organic and conventional is narrowing. "In some cases, it's almost neck and neck with conventional," he says. "For any school wanting to change to organic, costs would increase, but not as much as it would have ten years ago."

"FARM AT COLLEGE"

While farm to college is a growing trend, MUM's organic food program is best described as "farm at college." The university grows most of the vegetables served in its dining hall.

In 2003, the university started an organic farming project to provide fresh vegetables to students. The project, led by directors Tom and Kathy Brooks and Steve McLaskey, features a one-acre greenhouse, two smaller greenhouses, a seven-acre vegetable field, and an orchard of fruit trees and plants.

MUM's farm produces more than sixty varieties of vegetables and fruits, including beans, broccoli, carrots, cucumbers, leafy greens, such as collards, kale, and salad mixes, potatoes, spinach, sprouts, squashes, such as zucchini, yellow and winter tomatoes, and watermelons. They even grow edible flowers, such as nasturtiums.

Production is year-round, with some vegetables, such as leafy greens, grown during the winter in the heated greenhouses.

Vegetables are often picked and served the same day. "There's no comparison with regards to freshness," says Siegel.

The farm supplies about 80 percent, about 3,000 pounds per week, of vegetables used by MUM food service in July, August, and September and about one-third the rest of the year.

McLaskey, who has a doctorate in horticulture from Cornell, says the goal is to supply 100 percent of the kitchen's needs year round. "We want to produce the freshest and highest quality food possible," he says.

COLLEGE ORGANIC FARMS

Similar organic farming projects have sprouted at some forty colleges and universities, including Cornell, Rutgers, Michigan State, Iowa State, New Mexico State, University of Vermont, and the University of California.

The schools offer courses in organic agriculture, along with hands-on experience working on schools' farms. MUM students taking such courses spend half the day studying in the classroom and the other half working in the fields.

Organic food and farming programs at schools and colleges are cultivating a new generation of students who appreciate and value organic and locally produced foods. The programs offer students the ideals of organic and sustainable agriculture and provide healthier food. They support a respect for the environment, an appreciation of family farms, and a vision of life as an integrated whole.

As a result, students like Nicole Windenberger are likely to live and express these ideals throughout their lives, which will contribute to a better world. After graduation, Windenberger plans to go into sustainable consulting or education, for example teaching young people about organic agriculture, renewable energy, and "green" building, as she is learning. She says her education has been "about making my own life more sustainable. I will carry it through the rest of my life."

Chapter 9

ORGANIC
BIG AND SMALL

It's hard to imagine two organic farmers more different than Eliot Coleman and Gene Kahn. They even work on opposite ends of the United States. Coleman has farmed organically in Maine for more than thirty years. He grows fruits and vegetables year-round, no small feat in Maine, and sells them locally. Coleman's pioneering work has inspired thousands of organic farmers and gardeners. Three thousand miles west in Sedro Wooley, Washington, Gene Kahn grew Cascadian Farms from a small hippie organic farm in the early 1970s to a leading organic food brand. In 1999, Kahn sold his company to General Mills, where he is now a vice president.

While Coleman believes organic farming is meant for small-scale, diverse production that provides fresh, wholesome food to local populations, Kahn aims to bring organic food to the general public using large-scale farming techniques.

IS SMALL BEAUTIFUL OR BIGGER BETTER?

Within the organic movement, an internal divide has opened between proponents of small-scale organic farms selling locally like Eliot Coleman, and those who want to bring organic to the masses like Gene Kahn.

Devotees of the small-is-beautiful organic theory say big organic overextends the ecological functioning of an organic system by using crop monocultures, synthetic ingredients and inputs, long-distance transportation, and other troubling aspects of industrial food production. Those subscribing to the bigger-is-better philosophy say organic must increase in size to attract more consumers, and it can do so without compromising the organic ideals. Otherwise, as Gene Kahn says, organic will remain high-priced "yuppie food."

"PIONEERS ATTRACT SETTLERS"

Big organic is definitely a trend. Major food companies, attracted by organic foods' annual 20 percent growth, have either purchased organic companies or launched their own organic brands. General Mills's purchase of Gene Kahn's Cascadian Farms is one example. Dean Foods, one of the nation's leading dairy producers, owns White Wave, maker of Silk organic soymilk, and Horizon Organic Dairy. Kellogg Company owns Kashi, producer of natural and organic cereals. Coca Cola owns Odwalla, a natural juice manufacturer. Kraft Foods owns Boca Burger and Back to Nature Foods. M&M/Mars owns Seeds of Change, a leading producer of organic seed. H.J. Heinz owns a 20 percent share of Hain-Celestial, which owns more than a dozen organic/natural food brands. Heinz launched an organic version of its venerable ketchup. Campbell Soup Company sells organic soups and tomato juice. Domino sells organic sugar. Frito-Lay sells corn chips made with organic corn.

"It is only natural that as the industry grows, it attracts big companies. Pioneers attract settlers," says George Siemon, chief executive officer, Organic Valley Family of Farms.

Gene Kahn argues that the transition from small to big is necessary. "There's been a transition from a movement to a business. You have to play by the rules of the food business. It doesn't mean we'll lose our soul or the meaning of organic. Rather, it's the chance to have a much greater presence," he says.

Eliot Coleman disagrees. "The only organic companies that have been bought out are those whose quality is so dubious you don't want to buy their food no matter how many times they can legally print the word 'organic' on the label," he writes. Coleman says he would not even use organic Wheaties as compost.

CHALLENGES WITH BIG ORGANIC

There have been problems with big organic. Shortly after the U.S. Department of Agriculture's National Organic Program (NOP) rules became law in 2002, Fieldale Farms Corp., a large Georgia-based poultry company, attempted to overturn the rule requiring the use of organic feed in organic meat and dairy production. The company got its congressman, Nathan Deal, to slip a provision, or rider, into a

3,000-page congressional spending bill that would override the requirement for organic feed if a government study found that organic feed costs twice as much as nonorganic. The *St. Petersburg Times* described the attempt to change the rules as "a sleazy political favor." The organic industry, backed by other members of congress, reacted with outrage, and the rider was later overturned.

In 2005, the Wisconsin-based Cornucopia Institute, an organic watchdog group, filed a complaint with the USDA charging that Horizon Organic Dairy and Aurora Farms, two large organic dairy companies, abused rules recommending that dairy cows be allowed to graze on pasture. The group claimed the two companies confined their cows in feedlots, giving them little or no access to pasture. In contrast, small organic dairy farms graze cows on pasture, which the organic rules prescribe.

Mark Kastel, senior farm policy analyst at the Cornucopia Institute, said Horizon and Aurora operated their businesses like industrial-conventional dairy productions. "It's asinine to say they are organic farmers," he said. "You could say this is a fraud. Consumers aren't getting what they paid for."

The complaint led the National Organic Standards Board to recommend tightening rules requiring that cows raised to produce organic milk be grazed on pasture.

In addition, some big companies import organic crops from outside the United States to cut costs, which hurts markets for American organic farmers. White Wave imports organic soybeans from China, Brazil, and Argentina because it says there are not enough supplies in the United States. Cascadian Farms now buys many of its fruits and vegetables from Mexico, China, New Zealand, and Chile. By purchasing imports, these companies are not supporting the growth of organic farming in the United States.

Harvey v. USDA

In 2002, another small-scale Maine organic farmer, Arthur Harvey, threw a gigantic wrench into the Big Organic works when he filed a lawsuit against the USDA claiming that the NOP rules violated the Organic Foods Production Act of 1990 (OFPA), the congressional act that created the rules. In 2005, a federal district court ruled in Harvey's favor on three counts. In one count, the court said that the use of thirty-eight synthetic ingredients, which the NOP had approved for use in products labeled "organic," was inconsistent with OFPA and should not be allowed.

The allowance for synthetic ingredients, which increase shelf life, ease of shipping, and storage, has allowed big companies to produce organic cookies, crackers, cereals, and even TV dinners. Gene Kahn, who was an early member of the National Organic Standards Board, lobbied hard to allow the use of synthetics.

But many in the organic movement agree with Fred Kirschenmann, executive director of the Leopold Center for Sustainable Agriculture, who says synthetics are "contrary to the ecological principles of organic food production." The *Harvey* trial rulings would have forced the USDA to prohibit the use of synthetics in organic products. But the Organic Trade Association (OTA) led a successful effort to persuade Congress to amend OFPA and allow the continued use of synthetics, a move that overrode the court's rulings.

OTA's action produced a flood of criticism from consumer and public interest groups and other organic supporters. These concerned citizens called OTA's move a "sneak attack" that would allow the USDA to weaken the organic rules. OTA countered by claiming that its action was necessary because the *Harvey* rulings would have damaged the organic industry by severely reducing the number of organic products, which then would have ruined markets for organic farmers' crops.

Still, a few organic leaders criticized OTA's action. Jim Riddle, chairman of the National Organic Standards Board at the time, called the OTA-led rider a "flawed proposal." In particular, many expressed concerns over an "emergency procedure" amendment that would allow the agriculture secretary to approve the use of more synthetic ingredients if organic alternatives are not available due to a natural disaster.

The *Harvey* lawsuit and its aftermath left the organic community even further divided between proponents of big and small organic, a situation that does not bode well for the future of organics.

ALTERNATIVES TO "ORGANIC"

Much of the small versus big argument focuses on the NOP rules. Supporters of the NOP say the rules are the best in the world and that they give consumers a consistent meaning to the term "organic." Others say the rules favor big companies.

As a result, Eliot Coleman and other small organic proponents have opted out of organic certification completely. Coleman believes that food produced using sustainable farming methods and sold locally is "beyond organic" and should carry a separate distinction, which he describes as "authentic." Coleman writes, "'Authentic' is meant to be the flexible term 'organic' once was. It identifies fresh foods produced by local growers who want to focus on what they are doing, instead of what they aren't doing." In California, Rick and Kristie Knoll, owners of Knoll Farms, also dropped organic certification and are now using the word "tairwa," which is derived from the French word, "terroir," meaning "the essence of the land."

UPHOLDING THE STANDARDS IS KEY

Despite the challenges with big organic, some organic movement leaders say the entrance of the big companies is positive. "They are playing by the rules," says Organic Valley CEO Siemon. "They have no interest in challenging the integrity of organics because they will be scrutinized."

Even Kastel, from the Cornucopia Institute, admits some big companies uphold the organic standards. He points to H.J. Heinz, which purchases organic tomatoes from small organic farmers for its organic ketchup and proudly labels its branded product as organic. "It's a good example of someone doing it right," he says. Jim Riddle says organic food producers of all sizes are needed. "Farmers need the markets regardless of whether they're selling to General Mills or a small miller," he says. "There is room for large and small."

The big versus small debate may be a healthy sign that the organic movement can encompass very different viewpoints, such as those of Eliot Coleman and Gene Kahn. Perhaps the tension between the viewpoints will help refine the organic rules and push the movement toward greater growth or, as was seen in the *Harvey* lawsuit controversy, the differences could tear it apart.

Ultimately, what should unite organic supporters is a commitment to preserve the basic standards of the organic food movement. These standards require working with natural systems, protecting and preserving soils, plants, and water, using only materials and ingredients that do not harm life, and treating animals humanely. The standards ensure that organic farmers and food manufacturers produce foods that sustain human beings and the environment. One can argue these standards are vital to preserving life on Earth. Maintaining and defending the integrity of these standards in the face of government and big organic attempts to degrade them is the foremost responsibility of everyone in the organic community. Otherwise, as a *New York Times* editorial titled "Organic Drift" stated, "unless consumers can be certain that those [organic] standards are strictly upheld, 'organic' will become meaningless."

Chapter 10

THE BOTTOM LINE

*The food we choose has an impact upon the lives of other people,
upon the earth, and upon the future of humanity.*

—John Ikerd, professor emeritus of agricultural economics,
University of Missouri

One of the biggest complaints about organic food is its cost. It does cost more than conventional food, generally as much as 20 to 50 percent more, depending on the season and availability of a product.

WHY ORGANIC COSTS MORE

Organic farmers must meet strict standards for organic certification, which requires additional time, labor, and management costs. For example, they must document every step of production to verify compliance with the National Organic Program rules. Organic farmers and organic food companies must also pay to be certified.

Organic farming requires more labor. The farms tend to be small, and many tasks, such as weeding and harvesting, are done by hand.

Because organic food is produced on a smaller scale, it lacks the economies of scale that allow big food companies to purchase large quantities of crops or ingredients at low prices. The conventional food production system is designed to handle large volumes of just a few agriculture products. With its diversity and smaller volumes, organic does not fit into this system, resulting in added costs for transportation, distribution, and processing. For example, organic farmers generally harvest smaller volumes, so transportation companies may have to make multiple stops to pick up crops from several farmers, as opposed to making one stop at a large conventional farm. Also, organic food manufacturers purchase smaller amounts of specialty grains or ingredients, which cost more.

Unlike conventional farmers, organic farmers do not receive government subsidy payments to support their efforts. Without these subsidies, many conventional farmers would go out of business because prices paid for commodity crops, such as corn, soybeans, and cotton, are very low. In 2005, farm subsidy payments totaled more than $22 billion. In addition, organic farmers receive little government support for organic agriculture research. The U.S. Department of Agriculture devotes just 0.1 percent of its research budget to organic agriculture.

FARMERS NOT GETTING RICH

Like everyone else, organic farmers need to be paid fairly to remain in business. They follow strict certification rules to ensure that consumers receive a quality product. It is only fair that they receive adequate compensation. At the same time, despite the higher prices, it is safe to say that organic farmers are not becoming rich from their work.

Leaders of the organic food movement aim to reduce organic food prices. "This movement did not start out to establish expensive, niche-market foods for rich people but to model an alternative system for all of agriculture. We must make this accessible for all people," says Michael Sligh, director of the sustainable agriculture program Rural Advancement Foundation International-USA.

THE REAL COSTS OF "CHEAP FOOD"

When comparing the price of organic with conventional food, the main question to ask is not, "Why does organic cost more?" but "Is conventional food really cheaper?" We often hear that America has the cheapest food in the world. From a narrow perspective this may be true, but when looking at the big picture it is not.

Conventional food production is designed to produce the most food at the cheapest prices. This is achieved through massive monocultures of grains and vegetables, heavy doses of chemical pesticides and fertilizers, intensive processing to make foods last longer, and long-distance transportation. All these are direct costs.

But what about the indirect, hidden costs we consumers don't see on our grocery bill but pay for later? The costs are passed along to nature to absorb in the form of waterways polluted by agricultural chemicals and factory farm animal manure and the erosion of soil. Nature must be cleaned up and renewed. There are costs passed along to individuals, families, and loved ones who pay with pesticide-related illnesses and death. And what about the costs passed along to society, which has to absorb increasingly expensive fuel needed to power farm machinery, make chemical fertilizers and pesticides, and transport food thousands of miles? Organics is farm-by-farm, community-by-community closing this wild-ended logic with a sum that is far more beneficial than its parts.

When calculating the true cost of conventional food, these hidden costs must be included:

- Billions of dollars in healthcare costs to treat 76 million cases of foodborne illness each year, which result in 5,000 deaths and the acute pesticide poisoning of 300,000 farm workers every year

- The annual cost of obesity, $75 billion, which is twice as large as the fast-food industry's total revenues

- Uncalculated economic and social losses due to the growth of massive factory farms, which drive millions of farmers off the land, resulting in the loss of thousands of rural communities

- The negative environmental impacts of conventional agriculture cost between $5.7 and $16.9 billion per year, according to Iowa State University economists

- More than $20 billion in government farm subsidies paid each year to put "cheap" food on America's dinner plates

Taxpayers often foot the bill for government subsidies. When all of these hidden, indirect costs are added, America's cheap food becomes a whole lot more expensive. Moreover, organic food production would help eliminate many of these costs. For example, organic farming's prohibition of toxic pesticides would help clean up waterways, protect farm workers' health, and reduce incidences of pesticide-related illnesses. Local food production would save millions in food transportation costs.

CHOOSING ORGANIC

People can choose to buy "cheap" conventional food with its hidden costs, or they can choose food that enhances human health and preserves the environment. The majority of consumers, unaware of the problems with conventional food production and its hidden costs, choose the former. But an increasing number of people choose the latter.

They perceive greater value in organic. The old saying, "you get what you pay for" applies. With organic, consumers obtain food produced to the highest standards of quality and purity. As discussed in Chapter 6, scientific research is just beginning to show the nutritional advantages of organic food.

In addition, buying organic impacts the world beyond the individual, rippling through agriculture, the environment, health care, and the economy. People who buy organic support a system of agriculture that enriches the soil, protects and conserves water resources, and promotes biodiversity. They help reduce the amount of toxic pesticides that pollute waterways and harm human health. They reject the hazards of genetically altered food. They help stop the increasing domination over food by a few multi-national companies. They help keep farmers on the land, saving family farms and preserving rural communities.

People create an even greater impact by buying *local* organic. Local purchases reduce the amount of transportation needed to ship food, which means there is less oil consumption and air pollution. Local organic purchases support local farmers, keeping them in business, and support the regional economies of towns, cities, and states. Local organic purchases also protect consumers against increasing hazards of centralized industrial agriculture, such as foodborne illnesses.

People do make a difference with their food choices. The small ripples created by individuals choosing organic is rising to a tidal wave of change that will transform agriculture and food production, resulting in better human health, a cleaner environment, vital farming communities, a more balanced economy, a greater appreciation for how food is produced, and a renewed connection between farmers and consumers.

BUYING ORGANIC

There has never been a better time to buy organic food. Consumers will find more options, many buying outlets, and frequent opportunities to pay as little as, or even less than, the cost of conventional food.

In the past, people who wanted to buy organic shopped at natural food stores, which were few and far between. Today, organic consumers can shop at large natural food chains, such as Whole Foods and Wild Oats; gourmet-type food stores, such as Trader Joe's; independent natural food stores and cooperatives; conventional supermarkets; farmers markets; community supported agriculture (CSA) programs; buying clubs; and the Internet. There are even organic food home delivery services in some areas.

12 TIPS FOR BUYING ORGANIC

Here are some tips for buying organic:

1. **Evaluate your food budget to make room for organic.** Examine your weekly or monthly food purchases and see which conventional or fast foods can be dropped in favor of competitively priced organic items.

2. **Start by buying organic alternatives to one or two of the foods you eat the most.** Set priorities on what organic foods you want to eat. You can then add items as cost and availability allow. For example, many mothers are concerned about the use of genetically engineered bovine growth hormone (rBGH) in milk production and buy organic milk for their children instead.

3. **Look for and learn to read the organic label.** Foods are labeled organic according to the percentage of organic content, either 100 percent, 95 percent, 70 percent, or less than 70 percent (see Chapter 4). Be wary of foods labeled "natural." The natural label can be

misleading because, unlike organic, there are no rules for labeling foods natural. As a result, products can be labeled "natural" even though there is nothing natural about them.

4. **Shop at farmers markets.** The number of farmers markets in the United States is increasing dramatically, and there are good reasons for this. Farmers markets can offer the freshest, best-tasting organic fruits and vegetables at the best prices (see Table 11.1). Some farmers that sell at farmers markets may not be certified organic, but in general they use either organic or sustainable methods that do not involve the use of chemical pesticides. To find a farmers market near you visit www.localharvest.org, www.ams. usda.gov/farmersmarkets, or www.foodroutes.org.

5. **Join a community supported agriculture (CSA) program.** This is another excellent way to buy locally grown organic foods at reasonable prices. As described in Chapter 7, CSA members pay a subscription fee to a local farmer in return for weekly deliveries of fresh organic produce throughout the growing season. In addition, both farmers markets and CSA programs often offer rare heirloom fruits and vegetables that are never sold in stores. For more information, visit www.nal.usda.gov/afsic/csa, www.localharvest.org, or www.foodroutes.org.

6. **Join a natural food co-op or buying club.** Food cooperatives are member- or customer-owned businesses that provide quality food products to their members. Co-ops obtain volume discounts on food purchases and pass these on to members. There are more than 300 natural food co-ops in the United States. To find a co-op near you, visit www.coopdirectory.org.

   Food buying clubs consist of a few individuals who join together to buy organic foods directly from a large distributor. Buying club members can save as much as 30 to 40 percent off retail prices.

7. **Choose organic fruits and vegetables over conventional counterparts that are known to have high levels of pesticide residues.** These include apples, bell peppers, celery, cherries, chili peppers, imported grapes, nectarines, peaches, pears, raspberries, strawberries, and tomatoes. Organic apples are often competitively priced

with conventional apples. Other items may be competitively priced depending on the season.

8. **Buy items in bulk.** Purchasing bulk quantities of organic grains, beans, flour, dried fruits, and nuts costs less than packaged or canned. Many natural food stores and co-ops feature bulk sections.

9. **Buy organic fruits and vegetables when they are in season.** This allows you to get the best prices on the freshest organic fruits and vegetables. Organic produce sold out of season is likely to cost much more and be less fresh because it will have been shipped long distances. For example, zucchini sold in a suburban New Jersey Acme supermarket in November costs $7.98 per pound, while organic zucchini sold at an Iowa farmers market in June cost $1.00 per pound. You can find in-season organic produce at farmers markets and through CSA programs, natural food stores and co-ops, and conventional supermarkets.

10. **Buy "house" brands.** Natural and conventional retail grocery chains offer their own brands of organic products, which cost less than organic brands (see Table 11.1). Natural food retailers offering house brands include Whole Foods, Wild Oats, and Trader Joe's. Supermarket house brands include Safeway's Select and Kroger's Naturally Preferred, while Hy-Vee in the Midwest has Health Market, Giant Foods in the Mid-Atlantic offers Nature's Promise, and Publix in the South offers GreenWise.

11. **Shop around and look for bargains.** See which stores offer the best prices on organic. Most natural food stores and supermarkets will offer discounts or coupons for organic foods. For example, Stonyfield Farm offers $30 in coupons on its website, www.stonyfield.com, to purchase organic yogurt.

12. **Be creative.** Like organic raisin bran but not the price? Buy a plain organic whole grain cereal and add your own raisins. Make your own trail mix by buying organic fruits and nuts.

PLANT A GARDEN

You can take matters into your own hands and grow your own organic food in a garden. Gardening is a great hobby, nourishing to the body, mind, and soil. There is nothing better than garden-fresh fruits and vegetables. The only costs are the seed, your tender loving care, and a little sweat.

You can also participate in community gardens or urban agriculture projects that are sprouting nationwide. Urban gardens allow city dwellers to dig in and enjoy the benefits of locally grown organic food. For more information, visit www.greentreks.org/allprograms/rough terrain/urban gardening/index.asp or www.cityfarmer.org.

COMPARING CONVENTIONAL AND ORGANIC PRICES

As mentioned earlier, organic generally costs from 20 to 25 percent more than conventional food, but the conscientious shopper can find lower priced options. Shoppers are likely to find a range of price differences, as seen in Table 11.1, with some organic items costing less than conventional while some cost substantially more. For example, store brand organic oat bran cereal and corn chips cost less than conventional name brands, while prices for organic yogurt and pasta sauce are identical to conventional. Some items, such as apples, tomatoes, tomato juice, and fruit spread, cost just less than conventional, and others, such as potatoes, eggs, milk, and cereal, cost substantially more. These prices will range depending on the region of the country, the store, season, and product availability. As seen in Table 11.2, the best prices are often found at farmers markets. As with anything else, it's best to shop around to find the best prices.

TABLE 11.1. PRICE COMPARISON BETWEEN ORGANIC AND CONVENTIONAL FOODS*		
Food Item	**Conventional Price**	**Organic Price**
Apples (Red Delicious)	$.99 per pound	$1.35 per pound
Butter	$3.57 per pound	$4.99 per pound
Carrots	$.88 for 2 pounds	$1.89 for 2 pounds
Corn Chips	$3.29 for 12 ounces (Tostitos)	$2.19 for 13.5 ounces (store brand)
Eggs	$.83 per dozen	$2.29 per dozen
Fruit Spread	$2.39 for 10 ounces (Smuckers)	$2.99 for 10 ounces (Cascadian Farms)

Food Item	Conventional Price	Organic Price
Ketchup (Heinz)	$1.43 for 24 ounces	$1.99 for 15 ounces
Milk	$1.84 for half gallon	$3.25 for half gallon
Oat Bran Cereal	$4.19 for 15.7 ounces (Quaker Oats)	$2.29 for 15.7 ounces (store brand)
Pasta Sauce (Ragu)	$1.38 for 26 ounces	$1.38 for 26 ounces
Potatoes	$1.52 for 5 pounds	$4.99 for 5 pounds
Tomato Juice	$2.89 for 46 ounces (V8)	$3.19 for 46 ounces (Campbell's)
Tomatoes	$1.49 per pound	$2.15 per pound
Yogurt	$.79 for 6 ounces	$.79 for 6 ounces
Zucchini	$.99 per pound	$1.95 per pound

* Prices as they appeared in Everybody's Whole Food Store and Hy-Vee supermarket, Fairfield, Iowa, June 2005

TABLE 11.2. PRICE COMPARISON OF ORGANIC FOODS SOLD AT NATURAL FOOD STORE AND FARMERS MARKET*		
Food Item	**Natural Food Store**	**Farmers Market****
Broccoli	$3.29 per bunch	$1.00 per head
Cherry tomatoes	$1.59 for 1 pint	$1.25 for 1 pint
Eggs	$2.29 per dozen	$.75 to $1.00 per dozen
Radishes	$2.29 per bunch	$1.00 per bunch
Snow peas	$5.05 per pound	$2.50 per pound
Strawberries	$4.15 per quart	$2.50 to $4.00 per quart
Tomatoes	$2.15 per pound	$1.50 per pound
Zucchini	$1.95 per pound	$1.00 per pound

* Prices as they appeared in Everybody's Whole Food Store and a farmers market in Fairfield, Iowa, June 2005

** Items may not be certified organic, but are grown using organic methods or without pesticides

RESOURCES

Books

Fast Food Nation by Eric Schlosser (Houghton Mifflin, 2002)

Fatal Harvest: The Tragedy of Industrial Agriculture, edited by Andrew Kimbrell (Island Press, 2002)

Genetically Altered Foods and Your Health by Ken Roseboro (Basic Health Publications, 2004)

The New Organic Grower by Eliot Coleman (Chelsea Green Publishing, 1995)

Websites

FoodNews
www.foodnews.org/reportcard.php
Provides information on which fruits and vegetables contain the highest and lowest amounts of pesticide residues.

Food Routes
www.foodroutes.org
Provides resources for buying local food.

Local Harvest
www.localharvest.org
Provides resources for buying local food. Includes lists of farmers markets, community supported agriculture, food co-ops, and restaurants.

Organic Consumers Association
www.organicconsumers.org
Advocacy group for organic consumers. Provides information about organic foods.

Organic Trade Association
www.ota.com
Trade organization for organic farmers and food companies. Provides information about organic foods.

Seed Savers
www.seedsavers.org
Membership organization that saves and shares heirloom seeds from around the world.

Slow Food
www.slowfood.com
International association that aims to protect the pleasures of the table from the homogenization of modern fast food and life. Slow Foods favors local food traditions and defends food and agricultural biodiversity worldwide.

Sustainable Table
www.sustainabletable.org/home
Describes sustainable food production.

REFERENCES

Chapter 1

Cowley, Jeffrey. "Certified Organic." *Newsweek* (September 30, 2002): 53.

Editor. "Organic Research." *The Organic Report* (July 2004): 10Editor. "OTA Survey: U.S. Organic Sales Reach $10.8 Billion." *What's News in Organic* (July 2004): 1.

Editor. "A World of News." *What's News in Organic* (Spring 2006): 2.

The Hartman Group. "Organic2006: Consumer Attitudes & Behavior Five Years Later & Into the Future." www.hartman-group.com/products/studyOrganic2006. html. May 2006.

Howie, Michael. "Research Roots Out Myths Behind Buying Organic Foods." *Feedstuffs* (March 29, 2004): 19.

Organic Trade Association. "From Big to Small, Organic was the Hot Topic in Chicago." http://www.organicnewsroom.com/2006/05/from_big_to_small_organic_was.html. May 16, 2006.

United States Department of Agriculture Economic Research Service. "Organic Production, 1992–2003." www.ers.usda.gov/Data/Organic/index.htm.

Yussefi, M., H. Willer, B. Geier. "Organic Agriculture Worldwide." *IFOAM-Ecology and Farming* (January-April 2004): 12.

Chapter 2

Ackerman, Jennifer. "Food: How Safe?" *National Geographic* (May 2002): 2–31.

Cook, Christopher. *Diet for a Dead Planet.* New York, NY: New Press, 2004.

Delate, Kathleen. "Organic Agriculture." Iowa State University Extension brochure (May 2002): 2.

Environmental News Service. "Half the American Harvest Goes to Waste." November 23, 2004.

www.ens-newswire.com/ens/nov2004/2004-11-23-04.asp

Henry, Fran. "Breeding Contempt." *Cleveland Plain Dealer* (November 27, 2004).

Kimbrell, Andrew. *Fatal Harvest: The Tragedy of Industrial Agriculture.* Washington, DC: Island Press, 2002. 41, 52, 54,

King, Patricia. "Blaming It on Corn Syrup." *Los Angeles Times* (March 24, 2003).

Kuman, K., S.C. Gupta, et al. "Antibiotic Uptake by Plants from Soil Fertilized with Animal Manure." *Journal of Environmental Quality* Volume 34 (October 2005): 2082–2085.

Newman, Cathy. "Why Are We So Fat?" *National Geographic* (August 2004): 48.

Pollan, Michael. "Why Corn is King." *The New York Times* (July 19, 2002).

Schlosser, Eric. *Fast Food Nation: The Dark Side of the All-American Meal.* New York, NY: Houghton-Mifflin, 2001.

Stauber, John. "Statement of John Stauber on 2nd Confirmed Case of Mad Cow Disease." Organic Consumers website. www.organicconsumers.org/madcow/stauber062505.cfm. June 24, 2005.

Tilman, David; Fargione, Joseph; Wolf, Brian; Carla D'Antonio, Andrew Dobson, Robert Howarth, David Schindler, William H. Schlesinger, Daniel Simberloff, Deborah Swackhamer. "Forecasting Agriculturally Driven Global Environmental Change." *Science* Volume 292 (April 13, 2001): 281–284.

Tu, K. K. Donham, R., Ziegenhorn, et al. "A Control Study of the Physical and Mental Health of Residents Living Near a Large-Scale Swine Operation." *Journal of Agricultural Safety and Health* Volume 3(l): 13–26.

Wing, S. and S. Wolf. "Intensive Livestock Operations, Health and Quality of Life Among Eastern North Carolina Residents." *Environmental Health Perspectives* Volume 108 (2000): 233–238.

Chapter 3

Coleman, Eliot. *The New Organic Grower.* White River Junction, VT: Chelsea Green Publishing, 1995.

Gillman, Steve. *Organic Soil Fertility Management.* White River Junction, VT: Chelsea Green Publishing, 2002.

Reganold, J.P., J.D. Glover, et al. "Sustainability of Three Apple Production Systems." *Nature* Volume 410 (April 19, 2001): 926–930.

Uhland, Vicky. "Tapping the Heavens, Tilling the Earth." *Natural Foods Merchandiser* (September 2003): 36.

Vasilikiotis, Christos. "Can Organic Farming 'Feed the World'?" www.cnr.berkeley. edu/~christos/articles/cvorganicfarming.html. January, 26, 2005.

Zhu Y., H. Chen, et al. "Genetic Diversity and Disease Control in Rice." *Nature* (2000): 406, 718–722.

Chapter 4

Lambrecht, Bill. *Dinner at the New Gene Café.* New York, NY: St. Martin's Press, 2001.

National Center for Appropriate Technology (NCAT). "Organic Crops Workbook: A Guide to Sustainable and Allowed Practices." (October 2003): 32.

Chapter 5

Editor. "J.I. Rodale and the Rodale Family Celebrating 50 Years as Advocates for Sustainable Agriculture." *Pennsylvania's Environmental Heritage.* www.dep.state. pa.us/dep/PA_Env-Her/rodale_bio.htm (October 10, 1997).

Hepperly, P., R. Seidel, et al. "Water, Agriculture, and You." Kutztown, PA: The Rodale Institute, 2004.

Howard, Albert. *An Agricultural Testament.* Oxford, United Kingdom. Oxford University Press 1940.

Mergentine, Ken. "Organic Industry Roots Run Deep." *NFM's Organic Times* (1994): 63.

National Center for Appropriate Technology (NCAT). "Organic Crops Workbook: A Guide to Sustainable and Allowed Practices." (October 2003): 5.

Petersen, C., L.E. Drinkwater, et al. *The Rodale Institute Farming Systems Trial: The First Fifteen Years.* Kutztown, PA: The Rodale Institute, 1999.

Pimentel, D., P. Hepperly, et al. "Environmental, Energetic, and Economic Comparisons of Organic and Conventional Farming Systems." *BioScience* Vol. 55, No. 7 (July 2005): 573–582.

Rodale, Anthony. "The Rodale Vision Lives on Today." *The Organic Report* (July 2003): 34.

Chapter 6

Asami, D.K., Y. Hong, et al. "Comparison of the Total Phenolic and Ascorbic Acid Content of Freeze-Dried and Air-Dried Marionberry, Strawberry, and Corn Grown Using Conventional, Organic, and Sustainable Agricultural Practices." *Journal of Agricultural and Food Chemistry* Volume 51 (February 2003): 1237–1241.

Benbrook, Charles M. "Elevating Antioxidant Levels in Food Through Organic Farming and Food Processing." The Organic Center for Education and Promotion. January 2005.

Benbrook, Charles M. "Minimizing Pesticide Dietary Exposure Through Consumption of Organic Foods." The Organic Center for Education and Promotion. May 2004.

Curl, C.L., R.A. Fenske, et al. "Organophosphorus Pesticide Exposure of Urban and Suburban Pre-School Children with Organic and Conventional Diets." *Environmental Health Perspectives* Online. www.ewg.org/pdf/20021122_UWstudy. pdf. October 2002.

Ishida, B.K. and M.H. Chapman. "A Comparison of the Carotenoid Content and Total Antioxidant Activity in Catsup from Several Commercial Sources in the United States." *Journal of Agricultural and Food Chemistry.* Volume 52, Number 26 (December 29, 2004): 8017–8020.

Kimbrell, Andrew. *Fatal Harvest: The Tragedy of Industrial Agriculture.* Washington, DC: Island Press, 2002. 21.

Martens, Mary-Howell. "How Mary-Howell and Klaas Martens Made the Transition to Organic." *New Farm.* www.newfarm.org. August 2002.

Nielsen, Jacob H., Lund-Nielsen, Tina, Skibsted, Leif. DARCOF Enews, "Higher antioxidant content in organic milk than in conventional milk due to feeding strategy." www.darcof.dk. February, 19, 2005.

Porter, W.P., J.W. Jaeger, et al. "Endocrine, Immune, and Behavioral Effects of Aldicarb (Carbimate), Atrazine (Triazine), and Nitrate Fertilizer Mixture and Groundwater." *Toxicology and Industrial Health* Volume 15 (1999): 133–150.

Schafer, K.S., M. Reeves, et al. *Chemical Trespass: Pesticides in Our Bodies and Corporate Accountability.* San Francisco, CA: Pesticide Action Network North America, 2004.

Swan, S., C. Brazil, et al. "Geographic Differences in Semen Quality of Fertile U.S. Males." *Environmental Health Perspectives* Volume 111, Number 4 (April 2003): 414–420.

University of Rochester Medical Center, School of Medicine and Dentistry. "PCBS, Fungicide Open Brain Cells to Parkinson's Assault." www.urmc. rochester.edu/smd/ about/story.cfm?id=725. February 19, 2005.

U.S. General Accounting Office. "Agricultural Pesticides: Management Improvements Needed to Further Promote Integrated Pest Management." GAO-01-815 (August 2001): 4.

Chapter 7

Cantrell, Patty. "Family Farms Grow by Selling Shares to Neighbors." Michigan Land Use Institute. www.mlui.org/growthmanagement/fullarticle.asp?fileid= 16748. March, 20, 2005.

Choate, Mary S. "A Good Tomato in Winter, Where?" Co-op Food Stores website.

www.coopfoodstore.com/news/Archives/arch_nutatt/seasonal/tomatoes.htm l. July, 1 2005.

Filipic, Martha. "Interest Strong in Locally Grown Foods." Ohio State University Extension. www.ag.ohio-state.edu/~news/story.php?id=3002. April, 2, 2005.

Halweil, Brian. "The Farmers Market in Your Supermarket." *Organic Style* (February 2005): 34.

Pirog, R., T. Van Pelt, et al. "Food, Fuel, and Freeways: An Iowa Perspective on How Far Food Travels, Fuel Usage, and Greenhouse Gas Emissions." The Leopold Center for Sustainable Agriculture (June 2001): 2.

Pirog, R. "Ecolabel Value Assessment Phase II: Consumer Perceptions of Local Foods." The Leopold Center for Sustainable Agriculture (May 2004): 9.

Radice, Carol. "Produce Mantra: Think Globally, Source Locally." *Natural Foods Merchandiser* (March 2004): 88.

Roth, Cathy. "What is Community Supported Agriculture and How Does It Work? University of Massachusetts Extension. www.umassvegetable.org/food_farming_systems/csa/index.html. 6/15/06.

Spector, Rebecca. "Fully Integrated Food Systems." *Fatal Harvest: The Tragedy of Industrial Agriculture.* Washington, DC: Island Press, 2002.

Robyn Van En Center for CSA Resources. "What is Community Supported Agriculture?" Wilson College. www.wilson.edu/wilson/asp/content.asp?id=1273. 6/15/06

USDA-AMS Farmers Markets. "Farmers Market Growth." www.ams.usda.gov/farmersmarkets/FarmersMarketGrowth.htm. April 1, 2005.

Weise, Elizabeth. "Support from City Folk Takes Root on the Farm." *USA Today* (May 12, 2005).

Wilkins, Jennifer. "Think Globally, Eat Locally." *New York Times* (December 18, 2004).

Chapter 8

Budgar, Laurie. "Go Organic Dude." *Natural Food Merchandiser.* www.natural-foodsmerchandiser.com/ASP/1494/Display-Article. June 1, 2005.

Centers for Disease Control and Prevention (CDC). National Health and Nutrition Examination Survey (NHANES). As reported in "Successful Students Through Health Food Policies (SSTHFP)," California School Board Association and California Project Lean, 2003.

Muskus, Jeff. "Yale Seeks Increase in Organic Food." *Yale Daily News* (April 8, 2005).

Yale Sustainable Food Project. www.yale.edu/sustainablefood/garden.html. May, 25, 2005.

Chapter 9

Brasher, Philip. "Organic Food Producers Lose Ground to Imports." *The Des Moines Register* (October 8, 2005).

Coleman, Eliot. "Authentic Food-Authentic Farming." Four Season Farm. www.fourseasonfarm.com/main/authentic/beyond.html. April 2, 2005.

Coleman, Eliot. "Can Organics Save the Family Farm?" *Rake Magazine* (September 2004). www.rakemag.com/features/detail.asp?catID=61&itemID=19847

Editor. "Organic Drift." *New York Times* (November 4, 2005).

Meir, Tom. "Gene Kahn: Chicago-born Organic Pioneer Journeys from Hippie Farmer to Top Executive in Food Industry." *Conscious Choice* (March 2000). www.consciouschoice.com/2000/cc1303/genekahn1303.html.

Pollan, Michael. "Behind the Organic-Industrial Complex." *New York Times* (May 13, 2001).

Chapter 10

Editor. "When it pays to buy organic." *Consumer Reports.* (February 2006). 12.

Harrison, Christy. "Cost in Translation." *Grist Magazine* (August 25, 2005): www.grist.org/news/maindish/2005/08/25/harrison-organics/index.html.

Haumann, Barbara. "Buying for Organic: Considering the Real Costs." *What's News in Organic* (Nov/Dec. 2000): 1.

Kegans, Mark. "Mountains of Corn and a Sea of Farm Subsidies," *New York Times* (November 9, 2005).

Kimbrell, Andrew. *Fatal Harvest: The Tragedy of Industrial Agriculture.* Washington, DC: Island Press, 2002. 54.

Ikerd, John. "The High Cost of Cheap Food." *Small Farm Today* (July/August, 2001): www.ssu.missouri.edu/faculty/jikerd/papers/SFTcheapfood.html.

Schlosser, Eric. *Fast Food Nation: The Dark Side of the All American Meal.* New York, NY: Houghton Mifflin, 2002.

Sligh, Michael. "Organic at the Crossroads." *Fatal Harvest: The Tragedy of Industrial Agriculture.* Washington, DC: Island Press, 2002.

Tegtmeier, E.M. and M.D. Duffy. "External Costs of Agricultural Production in the United States." *International Journal of Agricultural Sustainability* Volume 1, Number 1 (2004): 1–20.

Chapter 11

Lazarony, Lucy. "17 Tips for Buying Organic Food on the Cheap." Bankrate www.bankrate.com/brm/news/cheap/20040901a1.asp. (2004): 104–105.

McCleary, Kathleen. "Organic Food for Less." *Organic Style* (May/June 2003): 128.

INDEX

ABOUT
THE AUTHOR

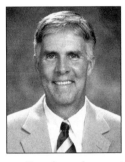 **Ken Roseboro** is editor and publisher of *The Non-GMO Report*, a monthly newsletter focusing on the risks of genetically engineered foods, and is the author of *Genetically Altered Foods and Your Health* (Basic Health Publications, 2004). He is also editor and publisher of *The Non-GMO Sourcebook*, an annual directory of suppliers of non-genetically engineered and organic seed, grains, ingredients, and foods.

Roseboro has written extensively about GE and organic foods for natural food industry publications, including *Natural Foods Merchandiser, Organic Processing, The Organic Report, Natural Products Industry Insider, Cooperative Grocer,* and others. He has also given presentations about GE foods and their impact on organic at tradeshows and conferences. Roseboro is also a certification committee member with an Iowa-based organic certification organization, as well as a member of the board of directors of the Iowa Organic Association.